P9-DZN-625

Family Care of
the Elderly

Family Care of the Elderly

Public Initiatives and Private Obligations

ST. JOSEPH'S UNIVERSITY

3 9353 00226 8934

Dwight L. Frankfather
The University of Chicago

Michael J. Smith
Hunter College

Francis G. Caro
Community Service Society
of New York

HV
1461
.F7

LexingtonBooks
D.C. Heath and Company
Lexington, Massachusetts
Toronto

242290

Library of Congress Cataloging in Publication Data

Frankfather, Dwight, 1946–
    Family care of the elderly.

    Includes index.
     1. Aged–Home care–United States. 2. Aged–Care and hygiene.
I. Smith, Michael J. II. Caro, Francis G., 1936–   . III. Title.
[DNLM: 1. Geriatrics. 2. Home nursing. 3. Social work. WT 100 F831f]
HV1461.F7   362.6'3   80–7577
ISBN 0–669–03759–1   AACR2

Copyright © 1981 by D.C. Heath and Company

All rights reserved. No part of this publication may be reproduced or trans-
mitted in any form or by any means, electronic or mechanical, including
photocopy, recording, or any information storage or retrieval system,
without permission in writing from the publisher.

Second printing, March 1984

Published simultaneously in Canada

Printed in the United States of America on acid-free paper

International Standard Book Number: 0–669–03759–1

Library of Congress Catalog Card Number: 80–7577

Contents

List of Figure
and Tables

Foreword

The evolution of the welfare state in the twentieth century has been accompanied by recurrent and exasperating contradictions, which are not new but troublesome. The research on which this book is based addresses four of these contradictions directly or indirectly: the character of the formal organization that deals with human distress; the relationship between the roles of family and bureaucracy; the function of professionalism; and the choice of suitable research methods. The research is based upon a small-scale program in one part of a major city and is circumscribed by the realities of studying a human-need-serving operation in vivo. Nonetheless, it opens important perspectives on the larger contradictions alluded to.

It is worth reexamining these contradictions in the light of this book, especially since the national election of 1980 has opened the door to a major recasting of the paradigm on which welfare evolution has proceeded since the 1930s. That paradigm included the beliefs that: a succession of group-identified needs warrants government action, action is benign and helpful, family life is enhanced by relief of onerous caretaking tasks, large-scale organization is efficient and responsive to human needs, professional skill is central to service delivery, research is most revealing when it is based on manipulation of quantitative data and an experimental rather than an observational model, and the objective in long-term care is an improved quality of life, which is ill defined. There seems to be a new paradigm replacing the old. The new one preserves the quantitative data preference but substitutes the following elements. Government effort to improve the quality of life, in social terms, is undesirable and not benign. Families should not be so substantially relieved of traditional caring tasks as in the past. Decision making and organization should be decentralized. Professionalism is possibly suspect and certainly overextended. It is against the background of this shift in thinking at the level of national government that this book can best be appreciated.

The most basic of the contradictions concerns our views about family obligation. On one hand, we believe in family integrity. We believe families should love and care for their members. But the economy, inflation, and contemporary views about personal or individual self-realization (for example, the freeing of women from the home) combine into an irresistible movement for able-bodied adults to work for wages. And this occurs at a time in human history when, for the first time, a significant proportion of the population lives into real old age—over sixty-five and into the seventy-, eighty-, and even ninety-year range. Although most of these elderly are physically competent during most of their later years, at least 20 percent will be so severely handicapped at any one time that they cannot perform major functions, and another 30 percent will be significantly limited. Family members still provide major physical care for their elders in almost all cases, but the volume of health and welfare services has also grown exponentially in real dollar terms in the past forty years. The old paradigm encouraged us to believe that even more should be done through formal arrangements and government means to improve the quality of life for all. The new paradigm encourages us to believe that too much has been done, that families have been "spoiled" and should reassume more of their traditional functions, and that our social services encourage families to substitute home-makers paid for by taxpayers for their own labors.

Finding a less-polarized and less-stereotyped position is not easy. Families and their personal circumstances are as varied as are the conditions of their dependent elders. The situation requires a sensitivity to families' capacities to do more than they do and an appreciation of how much families already do. An aging population brings new distress, which no civil society can or should ignore.

This leads naturally into the second contradiction, concerning the character of human-service organizations. These differ from most material-goods-producing enterprises in the almost infinite variety of conditions to be managed and the utmost subtlety and flexibility that delivery of decent service requires. The old paradigm recognized this only in part, but at least it encouraged many special-ized programs to evolve. The new one seeks to reduce variety and complexity and is derived from a citizen conviction that formal bureaucracies are unrespon-sive to their clients or consumers. The challenge under the old or the new ap-proach is how to make service delivery more rather than less responsive to users. Families can be the most flexibly responsive. They can be aware of and sensitive to the most subtle nuances of human need and adaptation—to erratic timing when help is needed and to unpredictable changes in condition. Even if a formal, bureaucratically organized staff cannot be quite as responsive as a family mem-ber because of a forty-hour, five-day work week, eligibility rules, case-load pressures, and malpractice liability, the challenge remains to make it more ac-ceptably responsive than is now the case.

In their analysis of the Family Support Program (FSP) and their subsequent proposals, the authors have offered several intriguing principles for making a service program more responsive to the needs of the disabled elderly population with family members. First they deal forthrightly with the issue of small volun-tary versus large public-service programs. The authors do so by matching the realities of fiscal limitations with the realities of long-term care burdens. Service decisions were based on a number of subjective judgments made either by family members or by service staff. A negotiated service contract depended on severity of disability, agreement among family members about the help they needed and their willingness to continue with their own support, and acceptance of conditions imposed by staff. Although this worked quite well, it also imposed serious stresses on both families and staff, especially as disability increased or family capacities deteriorated. The FSP model also was limited in its inability to handle large segments of the problem population, including those elderly who lacked family, whose relatives were distant, who could not agree on the support needed, or who were considered by staff to be unreliable or not capable of performing appointed tasks. The FSP was heavily dependent upon professional case diagnosis, selection, prescription, close monitoring, and rehabilitation directed at both the elderly and the family.

Within this framework, the FSP worked remarkably well by customary measures. A small staff with unrestricted though limited funds was able to supplement the caretaking of heavily burdened families, to control escalation of service demand, to keep ill elders in their accustomed environment, probably to delay nursing-home placement, and to do all this within cost levels comparable to or better than that of more restrictive services.

The authors present interesting and unusual evidence showing that many of the professional essentials on which FSP was based may be peripheral rather than central to the planning of major programs for the elderly. They also advance a maintenance model as being the major foundation for public policy rather than as one of several elements among which therapy, education, and rehabilitation dominate.

The maintenance-model proposals, insofar as they concern themselves with other organizational issues, provide general lines for public policy and for program developing in the future. After decades of categorical and specialized program building, it is both refreshing and disturbing to think about how the total population at risk could best be served, not in ideal or utopian terms but by organizationally responsive criteria. It may take a long time for the concepts advanced here to make their way into the consciousness of service organizers, professions, and policymakers. They are bound to have an influence, however, on the design of programs that can adapt equally well to the needs of the lone elderly, to those with caring families and those without, to various levels of disability, and to the preservation of life style, while minimizing administrative layers of control. Lest this be considered utopian, the proposal does not attempt to satisfy all wants; it does not seek to improve a vaguely articulated quality of life, whatever that may mean in specific cases. Instead it proposes a disability-entitlement benefit based on concrete and unambiguous measures of disability, full control over the use of the benefits by entitled beneficiaries, a client benefit account, staff accounting for the account draw-down, and staff information about optional uses. On balance, the proposed model fits well the American culture and the preferred way most persons choose to confront trouble: by personal choice and variation within accepted resource limitations. It also has the saving virtue of assuring much more flexibility to families than public policy now permits.

Such an organizational approach does not address the protective aspect of the subject directly. It assumes responsible behavior on the part of most persons, but protection against gross neglect or abuse for a few is missing or would require some other, more extraordinary approach. Here we confront a basic and unresolvable dilemma in complex society: just how far should society go to intervene to protect individuals, and against how much risk? A strong case can be made that for risk of injury only to oneself (falling or forgetting to take medication), choice is best left to the older person. The second line of protection should be the social pressure of one's peers, neighbors, and friends. This is made more difficult by the impersonal, sprawling, and mobile nature of modern life, but social regard of one's peers still has some force and is closer to the lives of most elderly than any bureaucracy can be. We may have a utopian vision that formal agencies can be superior to informal networks, but this vision is only imperfectly realized when informal networks collapse. Then the choice is for something in place of nothing. Finally, in cases of abuse and gross neglect, the courts remain as a final protection, which probably works no better or worse than social-service-organized protections.

A further question about the new approach is whether the market will produce the services wanted. Here the evidence is mixed, but if one sets aside questions of professional judgments about quality, the market has not worked too badly. Professionally controlled services like medical care have proven remarkably rigid in their adherence to an institutional and episodic medical-care format. Quality aside, proprietary home-care services have sprung up much more rapidly than have nonprofit, highly professionalized services. Proprietary nursing homes, with all their flaws, have developed rapidly to provide some care for the very sick aged when nonprofit homes for aged and agencies have lagged far behind. The caveat about the market in this field had best be considered moot until more work is done to test client satisfaction with a limited resource capacity to purchase what one wants.

In organizational terms, the question of the greater efficiency and sensitivity of small, nonprofit agency programs has also been explored. It is especially timely given the penchant of the new national administration for voluntarism over public service. The indirect costs for the FSP of about 50 percent of total costs is a possible but not yet proven characteristic of small service entities. If it is characteristic, it is a cost very difficult to justify except for experimental purposes. On the other hand, the administrative proportion of total costs of some very large public programs has also been estimated to run that high though not on a case-unit basis. Nonetheless, there is a surface logic to the claim that a personalized service, where staff and client work closely together, will be more sparing in the use of resources than will be a large, routinized system where clients can legally increase the draw-down to the limits of their benefits. Benefit levels may permit some beneficiaries to go beyond what they need to survive adequately.

The third set of contradictions has to do with the trend to professionalism in the human service and in the rest of American society (janitors are superintendents, undertakers are morticians, and so forth). Here the research is likely to raise a storm of protest from some professional quarters, but the argument should be out in the open and subject to more concrete scrutiny than has been true in the past. The key sticking point has to do with the place that counseling has in the constellation of essential services for the elderly. First it is necessary to clear away some obscuring underbrush. If counseling meant only sympathetic and sensitive encounters that clarify what a person wants and how it can be secured, there is no issue. But some professional doctrines have argued that clients are often unable to articulate their wants, and their requests only conceal deeper and more relevant needs. Similarly, applicants are said to be confused by their troubles and require discussion or aereation of emotion in order to function effectively. While there is no doubt that this is sometimes true, there is much doubt about how widespread this situation is and how counsel can best be provided.

This study is one of the rare few that has sought to give light without heat. It found that most clients did not recognize that they were getting a counseling service (they thought the worker was being friendly), but the workers thought they were giving a necessary amount of counsel and considered it a key part of their work. Social work literature in particular is strewn with observations to the same effect, and they have been generally ignored in shaping the profession. Studies of hospital social work consistently reveal that staff consider counseling their main professional task, whereas their daily duties (and expectations of their colleagues) consist of arranging a multiplicity of concrete services. Studies of early community action agencies in the war on poverty showed that most applicants came to agencies with one or two specific wants in mind whereas staff often considered that their wants concealed many other unexpressed needs that had to be explored.

None of this history argues that counseling is not a real and useful service. At issue is the relative place that counseling holds in relation to the many other functions that social workers perform. If the other, more-concrete functions make up a large part of the staff task, then they properly become the core or base for the profession to build on. Counseling need not be neglected, but it is no longer the measure of what is considered preferred practice, in emulation of psychiatry and psychology. At stake is the use of credentials and medical models on which to base a service profession, when other criteria, such as taking good care of a socially troublesome problem, might work just as well. The responsibility for this inverted scale of values rests on the current social value placed on high technology and science. The needs of the aged are more social than technical. It is difficult for an aspiring staff to take on a change in social values, but it is an unavoidable challenge.

In this most charged and emotional arena, the authors have produced tangible evidence, the interpretation of which can only be that if counseling is vital, then it should be made explicit to clients so that they know what they are getting. If this is done and confirms the profession's belief in that function, then client desire for it and willingness to pay for it will increase.

Finally, the research effort in human services is enormously enriched by the methodology used. After a few halcyon years of social work research, work with the aged has tended either to rely on manipulation of large masses of quantitative data, often drawn from national sampling, or to be satisfied with limited case observations and descriptions. In the 1970s when research funds were available for experimental purposes, the concern with numbers was augmented by a preoccupation with strictly experimental research design, which usually imposed so massive a research burden on early experimentation that both experiments and research foundered in inconclusiveness. In many instances, the cost of the evaluation component in new and untried demonstrations exceeded the investment in the service itself. This study demonstrates once again how valuable, and insight-enhancing, modest research can be if it is guided by a sure sense of proportion. In this case, the analysis of quantitative data (usually small numbers) has been clear, drawn from field trials but not trying to go beyond what a human field trial can tolerate at the first stage of tryout. This has been augmented by judicious and more valuable use of research, staff, and client observations, secured by interviews, and introduced into a narrative to give reality to other evidence. The result provides one of the best extant living pictures of what it means for families to take care of their sick elders; it shows what a service program can and cannot do. All this is disciplined by scrupulous attention to such quantitative data as could reasonably be extracted about the research questions posed.

At the end of this effort, many of the uncertainties in organization, family role, professional practice, and research method remain. But it is possible to view them in a less constricted, and much more pragmatic, humane manner. The policy and program suggestions lift the subject to a new plateau for testing, which is especially useful at a time of major national policy change toward human services. The approach suggested fits as well as anyone could expect for the twin needs of the elderly and the society in which they survive. This research into the nature and potential of professionalization in social welfare is given a set of conceptual and methodological tools that are not too confined by ideology or tradition.

Robert Morris
Brandeis University

Preface and Acknowledgments

Francis G. Caro

Providers of community-based service are accustomed to working with disabled older persons who strongly prefer to live independently, outside of an institution. At the same time, they encounter families who struggle to care for a disabled relative, become overextended, and seek professional assistance with institutional placement. The research and demonstration project we describe in this book attempted to establish a new collaborative arrangement between families and organized services. The purpose was to encourage family persistence and to sustain the independent living arrangements of disabled older persons. The project reflects a configuration of policy, service, and research interests. It provided an opportunity to address questions regarding the nature of the help provided by family members and the forms of help they would most welcome. It also permitted an exploration of the effects of introducing service on family members and on their community-care arrangements.

This program was conducted by the Community Service Society (CSS) of New York, one of the country's oldest and largest private, nonsectarian, social-welfare organizations. Both the demonstration services and the research were funded fully by the society between October 1976 and September 1979. The demonstration reflects a deliberate effort on the part of the society to integrate its research and direct-service efforts. By including researchers in the design and evaluation of service interventions, the society seeks to use its direct-service experience as a sound basis for informing professionals on issues concerning practice and public officials on underlying policy issues.

The demonstration was conducted within the framework of the Older Persons Service, a long-standing social casework unit serving the elderly and their families. When the society moved toward operating direct services within a demonstration context, the Older Persons Service staff was challenged to develop new strategies. The program described here is one of the new approaches that emerged.

The demonstration was named the Natural Supports Program. We have chosen instead to identify it here as the Family Support Program. Although it was more broadly conceived, the program, in fact, concentrated its efforts on assistance to relatives of the elderly disabled. At the risk of confusing professionals who know the program by its original name, we will use Family Support Program (FSP) in this book since it describes the demonstration more accurately.

This book is limited to reporting on the services provided by FSP on an individualized basis. We do not include an examination of a second group component of the society's program concerned with groups of families. There are substantial differences in the nature of the two strategies and limited overlap in the populations served. Because of its more intensive services, its importance for public policy, and the limited resources available for research, we decided to concentrate our research resources on the individual component.

This book is the report of researchers closely associated with FSP from the outset. The authors are associated with the Institute for Social Welfare Research, the Community Service Society's vehicle for conducting evaluation research and basic research on public-policy issues. At the time the program was conceived, the unit also had program-planning responsibilities. Although we played a major role in program design and regularly attended service staff meetings, our role in shaping the intervention was ultimately of an advisory nature. Decisions regarding the nature of the intervention were made by the service administrators and staff of FSP.

Dwight Frankfather prepared and supervised the research plan and authored the original program goals and procedures statements. Michael Smith assumed responsibility for managing the research component in the final year and was primarily responsible for assimilating the quantitative data for presentation. Frank Caro, as director of the research and evaluation office, assumed overall responsibility for the research. The three authors contributed equally to the book.

Although we were in agreement with our practitioner colleagues on many matters, we did have some important, persistent differences over service and policy priorities for FSP. A brief review of our differences will help to put the book in perspective. Methodologically, we recommended a staged approach to program implementation. We agreed with our colleagues that it was useful to initiate the programs on an exploratory basis so that inevitable implementation problems could be worked out on the basis of experience. When start-up problems had been solved, we proposed a second stage with more-formalized program procedures and a quasi-experimental or experimental design. For organizational reasons, the second stage did not materialize. Accordingly, both the service program and our research remained of an exploratory nature. Concerning research and policy preferences, we were unsuccessful in promoting the use of explicit criteria in accepting or rejecting service applicants. We also were unsuccessful in persuading the service staff to give applicants explicit information regarding the forms and scope of help they might expect. With neither sufficient funds nor a control- or comparison-group design, we lacked a strong base for testing hypotheses concerned with program effectiveness. In spite of these limitations, the service intervention did have innovative characteristics deserving research attention. Further, the program illuminates important, unresolved policy questions for community-based long-term care.

In preparing this book, we hoped to achieve balance in our presentation. We sought to provide an objective account of the demonstration, its clients, and their interaction with the program. We have depicted the program's contributions in illustrating the role that organized services can play in collaborating with families in community-based long-term care. We also introduced a critical policy perspective that reflects our commitment to rigorous standards for public programming.

The manuscript includes three major elements: (1) an analysis of issues involved in home care for the functionally disabled elderly, (2) an account of the experiences of the Family Support Demonstration, and (3) recommendations for public long-term care policy. In the final chapters, we outline an alternate model for a public entitlement program. In interpreting demonstration data and in discussing public-policy options, we present our own views. The public-policy recommendations are not necessarily those of the Community Service Society.

Acknowledgments

In a complex research-and-demonstration effort, it is impossible to acknowledge the contributions of all who played important roles. We appreciate the cooperation of the families with our research interviews. Both the demonstration program and the research enjoyed the support of CSS general directors Alvin Schorr and Bertram Beck. Myron (Mickey) Mayer showed persistent interest and gave encouragement as a representative of the CSS Committee on Aging, one of the society's major vehicles for lay participation. Robert Moroney of the University of North Carolina was an important source of help in shaping the program concept. When the program was introduced, Janet S. Sainer as director of CSS programs on aging played a key role in interpreting the program design to the direct-service staff. Program planner Susannah Gross-Andrew contributed a great deal to the service design and worked patiently with the service staff to resolve implementation problems. The FSP service director provided essential cooperation in many ways, including access to information regarding service transactions and comments on earlier versions of the research manuscript. The casework staff and social work students showed great patience in cooperating with data-collection requirements. Olivia Capers, Maureen Simone, and Denise Smith-Frasier served as research assistants. Olivia and Pat Ballard, from the service staff, deserve special notice for their unflappable styles and faithfulness to the principles underlying the venture. Betty Bradley, Helen McLaren, Helen Larmore, Edith Oxley, and Maren Grossman provided clerical assistance.

As manuscript editor and critic, Karen Peterson left few words unturned in her assiduous efforts to achieve a consistent style among the three authors.

Public Initiatives and Private Obligations

As public commitment to home care for the chronically impaired grows, the relationship between the family and the state takes on a new dimension of significance. Social definitions of responsibility for the chronically impaired are in transition. A new and more complex service alliance must reconcile the bureaucracy of the state with the informality of the family. In order for these two institutions to function harmoniously together, public programs must be clearly defined and carefully designed. The Family Support Project (FSP), a service demonstration and research project conducted by the Community Service Society (CSS) of New York, assisted families in maintaining their impaired elderly at home. The project was designed to explore the operational dimensions of the relationship. Participating family members described the supportive functions they performed and the services they needed, and the staff attempted to arrange flexible services that were compatible with the interests of both the family and the impaired person.

When family members provide services as diverse as the following, it is obvious that the realization of a meaningfully integrated contribution from formal organizations or public-service bureaucracies will be challenging:

> We put her in the shower and brush her teeth. . . . We put lipstick on her and put her hair in a french twist with floral combs. . . . When we go away overnight, we take her with us. . . . I put paper on the floor 'cause she doesn't always make it to the bathroom. . . . I'll paint her apartment, change the light bulbs, and wash the windows.

Not only the form but the allocation of responsibility is at issue. Will public programs replace family responsibility altogether? Will impaired elderly with families be singled out for reduced benefits or be made ineligible for all public home-care benefits? The social and economic costs of long-term care are high. In 1980, federal, state, and county governments spent $14 billion on such care. Families provided an equal or greater amount. Even a slight redistribution of responsibility for care will have a substantial effect on public costs and family burdens. Therefore the project also explored the persistence of the family in caring for the impaired and the extent of substitution once outside services were available.

The role of the family in maintaining dependent aged members is important, but it must be considered within the larger context of long-term care policy.

The parameters of this book are determined by currently debated policy questions about community-based long-term care.

Long-Term Care

Long-term care is a major service sector in which continued growth is expected. National statistics show that 80 to 85 percent of the aged have one or more chronic conditions.[1] Total private and public expenditures for long-term care rose from $12.5 billion in 1975 to an expected $26 billion to $31 billion by the end of 1980.[2] Demand will continue to grow with improved access to acute medical care for the aged, with increased longevity, and with a larger proportion of elderly in the population.

Federal funds for long-term care are distributed among an array of categorical federal, state, and local programs. Shea counted nineteen distinct programs.[3] Medicaid, Medicare, Title 20, Veterans Administration, Department of Housing and Urban Development, National Institute of Mental Health, and the Administration on Aging are all sources of public money for the purchase and delivery of care for the chronically disabled. Each program has separate rules, regulations, eligibility and benefit criteria, definition of service domain, standards for intensity of care, delivery mechanism, and administrative structures. Funds may flow from federal agencies directly to state agencies or local governments, through fiscal intermediaries to private facilities, and occasionally directly to the consumer. Although there are countless intersections among these programs, there is no centralization of structure or direction.

Approximately 90 percent of all public support for the chronically disabled goes for the purchase of institutional care (see table 1-1). The availability of institutional financing combined with the relative lack of home-care financing has channeled demand into the institutional sector. The ultimate distribution of service and dollars is a by-product of funding mechanisms rather than a response to demand.

This bias toward institutional care is thought to result in premature and unnecessary institutionalization. Either at public or private expense, many elderly receive a level of complete care seemingly unjustified by their slight or moderate impairments. Somewhere between 10 and 40 percent of the nursing-home population is receiving unnecessarily high levels of care.[4] Overutilization results in unnecessary costs. Nursing-home placement is also considered a less-desirable form of care because of the threat of isolation, depersonalization, loss of privacy, forfeiture of civil rights, unappealing social conditions, unappetizing meals, and public exposure of intimate family relations.[5] The absence of alternatives imposes this form of care on those unable to survive independently.[6]

Although medical care may be a relatively small proportion of the overall costs of maintaining the chronically impaired, the majority of existing programs

Table 1-1
Estimated Level of Public Support for Institutional and Home Care, 1975

Source	Support (millions)
Medicaid	
Institution	$4,330
Home	70
Subtotal	4,400
Medicare	
Institution	255
Home	185
Subtotal	440
Veterans Administration	
Institution	240
Home	5
Subtotal	245
SSI Supplemental payment (domiciliary care only)	40
Social services (home care only)	66
Total	
Institution	4,820
Home	326
Other state and local	
Institution	300–400
Home	230
Total public support	
Institution	5,145–5,205
Home	556

Source: Data from General Accounting Office, *Entering a Nursing Home—Cost Implications for Medicaid and the Elderly* (Washington, D.C.: Government Printing Office).

have been conceived and administered within the framework of the medical model. Medicare and Medicaid, the principal funding sources, are based on a health-insurance concept. Skilled nursing homes and intermediate-care facilities are modeled after hospital care. The medicalization of custodial, domestic, and social services creates confusion over the purpose of long-term care. The goal of medical intervention is rehabilitation and restoration of functioning, but long-term care by definition is directed at those for whom recovery is not expected. Ramifications of this confusion materialize in formulations of long-term care goals, technology, and administration.[7] Although concepts of maintenance and personal care are more-fitting alternatives to rehabilitation and treatment as underlying principles of long-term care, no profession is organized around a maintenance objective that could challenge the prior claims of the medical model and health professions. In chapter 7 a maintenance model is described that emphasizes user control, standardized eligibility and benefit criteria, and market incentives to expand service and contain production costs.

Nursing-home placement can be a convenient and simple solution to organizing services for the chronically disabled. Institutions combine in one setting a broad array of health, social, personal, and custodial care for the disabled. To public regulators, the performance of institutions is easier to monitor than that of dispersed individual providers. Hospital discharge staff members are not always aware of the few alternatives that do exist. They also prefer nursing-home placements when they are unsure about the quality and reliability of the options.[8]

The impaired elderly and their families are often unaware of their possible eligibility for alternative services.[9] Sometimes placement is the preferred option because organizing the necessary care in the community would require individual contracts with perhaps a dozen different service entities. The success of the package would depend upon the stability of the individual components, and rarely is one professional assigned to organize and monitor all of the components.

No administrative structure ensures proper accountability for all of the long-term care programs. Consumers and recipients of public benefits have little influence on the kind and quality of care. Even the definition of accountability is not well developed within the field of long-term care. Although there is much criticism over inappropriate levels of service, there is no agreement on the terms for recognizing or defining appropriate care.[10] Quality-assurance mechanisms and cost-control mechanisms have not been developed.

The public costs of various long-term care options are difficult to determine and predict. Per-capita and aggregate-cost comparisons across service strategies have not been made. Since greater numbers of seriously and chronically handicapped individuals are now living at home or with families than are residing in institutions, there is an enormous potential demand for noninstitutional care. The Congressional Budget Office estimates that 3.6 million to 7.8 million impaired aged are in need of services at home.[11] Even if home-care options reduced per-capita costs of care in the short and long run, aggregate demand would create a sizable budget expansion that would occur in the face of diminishing resources for public-service programs. Priorities must be established concerning whom to serve, when, and in what manner. There is a well-established tax base, as well as a private insurance industry, to underwrite medical and health care. There is no similar established revenue source for long-term care.

The Family

As far back as Victorian England, periodic hand-wringing has occurred over the increasing failure of families to care adequately for dependent children and the aged.[12] Since every generation produces such claims, nostalgia as much as changing patterns may explain the concern. It is difficult to detect autonomous change in a single variable when the context itself is shifting. Any change in family patterns is occurring simultaneously with increased longevity and greater disability, improvements in living standards, public provision of retirement income, health insurance for the aged, and new access to home care. Recent popular depictions of changes in family life now appear to be erroneous. For example, urbanization has not led to the anticipated spatial separation of the elderly from their children or to a reduction in frequency of contacts.[13] A national probability sample indicated that 77 percent of the aged had seen a child in the previous week, and 89 percent had done so in the previous month.[14] Solidarity and strong affectional bonds remain part of the modified extended family.[15]

The historical vision of the extended family in a single household no longer exists when different generations of a family prefer to live apart.[16] A pattern of multiple and independent subunits, however, is increasingly common. These nuclear subunits are not isolated but form a coalition of families in a state of partial dependence.[17] Whether this change affects the family's support of a chronically impaired member is difficult to determine. It is obvious that the possibility for functional assistance across family units is not exhausted, nor are more general forms of mutual aid and economic interdependence.[18]

In another popular stereotype, nursing-home placement is equated with abandonment, but available evidence contradicts this stereotype. Children who live within twenty-five miles of their parents in nursing homes are frequent visitors.[19] York and Calsyn reported that the mean number of family visits to nursing homes per month was twelve.[20] Even when families said that their visits were not always rewarding, they continued to visit frequently. Desirable effects on the emotional components of relationships among family members have been noted when nursing-home care was substituted for family care. Among these effects are reduced disruption to the occupational and familial roles of supporting family members, greater frequency of contacts, and improved respect, degree of expressed affection, and closeness among members.[21]

The availability of the family as a resource for long-term care, however, may be diminished by other contemporary and future changes. With a trend toward smaller families, parents with fewer children may have fewer support options in old age. As the divorce rates increase, more children may not acknowledge any obligation to their elderly parents and disregard them. As more women become employed outside the home and families rely increasingly on double incomes to maintain a desired standard of living, the adult daughter may not be available to provide support to dependent parents. Since the preponderance of home care is now provided by wives and daughters, the supply of family labor may diminish.[22] For the moment, however, a highly integrated, extended-family system survives that is capable of functionally supporting aged dependents. Many anticipate its continuing capacity to do so.[23]

There appears little doubt that the family currently is a significant source of care for the chronically disabled.[24] In Shanas's national probability sample, 3 percent of the noninstitutionalized elderly were bedfast and an additional 7 percent were homebound.[25] Both Shanas and Masciocchi observed that the family provides the bulk of home care to the seriously disabled community residents.[26] Brody estimates that 80 percent of all home health care is provided by the family.[27] Of those patients for whom personal care was prescribed upon discharge from a chronic hospital, 75 percent received that care from a family member.[28] And the more severe the impairment, the greater the families' contribution relative to all other agencies.

Numerous studies of nursing-home admissions also demonstrate the importance of family care in preventing nursing-home placement. Both Brody and Maddox conclude that the presence and the willingness of family members to provide care are the crucial factors in placement decisions.[29] Even across differential levels of disability, the family was the key variable.[30] Deterioration in the ability of the family to provide assistance leads to placement of the disabled. In the Townsend study, the most common events leading to institutionalization were the death or sudden illness of close family members.[31] Even the anticipation of loss of a close relative (through relocation, for example) encouraged some to seek admission. Cross-sectional comparisons of institutional and community residents provide further evidence that persons without close families are much more likely to be institutionalized. Although 6 percent of the aged were never married, 16 percent of those in nursing homes were never married.[32] When Masciocchi introduced level of disability into the comparison of characteristics, the role of the family appears more significant: "Two thirds of the non and mildly impaired aged in skilled nursing facilities had no family, nearly 80% severely and totally disabled in the community actually lived with family."[33]

Finally, from the perspective of the cost-conscious public sector, the families' persistence is an important substitute for nursing home and Medicaid financing.

Filial Obligation and Societal Transfers

The question remains whether the family or the state should bear the principal burden of responsibility for the seriously disabled aged. Historically the family has been the first line of responsibility for children and aged dependents. But these traditional family functions are transferred to the state when there is widespread failure of specific forms of private assistance or when the collective citizenry perceive some benefit. Society-wide transfers include health insurance, state mental hospitals, public education, housing, public health, income maintenance, social security, police protection, dog pounds, and national defense.

It appears there are adequate conceptual grounds for the transfer, whether partial or complete, of community-based long-term care responsibility to the public sector. The unpredictable occurrence of serious chronic impairment and the high cost of care may make family responsibility an onerous burden. Private resources are often modest and uncertain, and not all chronically impaired have families from which pooled support could come. Diamond reports that only 6 percent of nursing-home residents have families with incomes over $20,000.[34] Financially responsible relatives may have little to contribute from their incomes. Also, many children and siblings are in their early sixties and expect income reductions themselves in the near future.[35] In the Townsend study, 36 percent of the nursing-home admissions were living with relatives who were themselves ill or infirm.[36] Although some families are more solvent than others, the ability to purchase care from private income is beyond the means of most. Families experience income deficits and surpluses irregularly throughout the family life cycle and have difficulty in attempting to levy equitable sacrifices across generations.

Precedents for the assumption of public responsibility are already established. The old-age, social security concept could be extended to provide additional benefits to the disabled elderly. The Social Security Administration might become a direct provider in addition to distributing cash benefits.[37] Such a plan would establish long-term care in an insurance-based entitlement context. Public funds are already used extensively to purchase institutional long-term care. The Medicaid and Medicare payment mechanisms also establish an insurance-based entitlement context. Medicaid currently is funding numerous community-based long-term care demonstration programs.

It appears that the United States is moving gradually toward the provision of publicly financed, comprehensive long-term care within an entitlement framework, but full entitlement is not likely to be enthusiastically received at a time when economic conditions have reduced public resources for human services.[38] A public program that assured adequate solutions to the problems of daily living would be much less expensive if it could be limited to those without potential family caretakers. Therefore a two-tier approach may become a popular policy option. For seriously impaired persons without family resources, the state would assume complete service responsibility. For those with family resources, the state would offer a second tier of modest benefits with basic responsibility remaining explicitly with the family.

A program that attempts to serve all of the functionally disabled might have insufficient funding to provide adequate care for the seriously disabled without strong informal supports. In effect, those without family resources would remain at a disadvantage in their attempts to maintain residence in the community. Also the substitution of organized services for family-provided care may do little to improve the situation of the functionally disabled. The main effect may be to relieve family members.

Concentration of service resources on those without families, however, would provide an incentive for the dissolution of family care resources, that is, family ties may be severed to enable functionally disabled persons to qualify for publicly financed services. Instead a small compensation to families might be an adequate incentive for them to continue their support.[39] Perhaps benefits could be structured to keep public costs modest but sufficiently attractive to prevent artificial dissolution. The two-tier approach would also acknowledge that care-taking responsibility may be so great that the families deserve assistance.

In the past, eligibility criteria for entitlements have required contributions from beneficiaries and their families. Nursing-home residents were required to liquidate and exhaust their assets by the purchase of care from private means before becoming eligible for public financing through Medicaid. To become eligible for Medicaid, some nursing-home residents have transferred their assets to nonspouse family members, but Medicaid regulations permitted denial of eligibility when assets have been transferred. The considerable costs this policy imposes on heirs has provoked devious evasions and public outrage. Although some states maintain these eligibility requirements, many others have greatly tempered the definition of relative responsibility. In thirty-five states, Medicaid regulations are superseded by Supplemental Security Income (SSI) criteria, which do not restrict transfers and require spouse support only while the spouse is at home. One month after admission to a nursing home, the spouse at home is no longer responsible for contributing to the costs of care, regardless of financial resources. The emergence of relaxed asset-transfer criteria permits the inheritance of parental wealth, which indirectly reduces the cost of care to children. A policy that is prejudiced against chronically impaired elderly with families re-creates a practice that proved unpopular and unworkable when applied to nursing-home care. As long as Medicaid finances nursing-home care, family obligation for home care would be difficult to enforce. Anderson's analysis of Victorian English pension policy shows that attempts at compulsory mainte-nance by children made them bitter about giving aid. [40] In observing the historical parallel, Anderson wrote, "The constriction of non-institutional relief in England in the 19th Century for the purpose of encouraging thrift and family affection actually increased the workhouse population and diminished the possibility of small-scale exchanges of assistance among relatives."

Notes

1. See National Center for Health Services Research, *Elderly People: The Population 65 Years and Over,* DHEW Publication no. 77–1232 (Washington, D.C.: Government Printing Office, 1978).

2. Congressional Budget Office, *Long-Term Care for the Elderly and Disabled,* (Washington, D.C.: Government Printing Office, 1977).

3. John Shea, "Alternatives to Institutional Care," mimeographed (Chicago: Task Force for Alternatives to Institutional Care, Office of the Regional Director, Region V, DHEW, 1977).

4. Powell Lawton, "Institutions and Alternatives for Older People," *Health and Social Work* 3, no. 2 (1978): 123; Congressional Budget Office, *Long-Term Care*.

5. See Margaret Blenkner, "Social Work and Family Relationships in Later Life with Some Thoughts on Filial Maturity," in *Social Structure and the Family*, ed. Ethel Shanas and Gordon Strieb (Englewood Cliffs, N.J.: Prentice-Hall, 1965); William Bell, "Community Care for the Elderly," *Gerontologist*, 13, no. 3 (1973): 349–354; and Dwight Frankfather, *The Aged in the Community* (New York: Praeger Publishers, 1977).

6. Jane L. Barney, "The Prerogative of Choice in Long Term Care," *Gerontologist* 17, no. 4 (1977): 309–314.

7. William Pollak, *Expanding Health Benefits for the Elderly*. Vol. 1: *Long Term Care* (Washington, D.C.: Urban Institute, 1979).

8. Elaine Brody, "Long Term Care: The Decision-Making Process and Individual Assessment," in National Conference on Social Welfare, *Human Factors in Long-Term Care, Final Report of the Task Force*, 1975.

9. Susan Friedman et al., "Maximizing the Quality of Home Care Services for the Elderly," mimeographed (New York: Community Service Society, 1977).

10. Alan Sager, "Learning the Home Care Needs of the Elderly: Patient, Family and Professional Views of an Alternative to Institutionalization," mimeographed (Waltham, Mass.: Levinson Policy Institute, Brandeis University, 1979).

11. Congressional Budget Office, *Long-Term Care*; See also General Accounting Office, *Entering a Nursing Home—Costly Implications for Medicaid and the Elderly*, Report to the Congress (Washington, D.C.: Government Printing Office, November 26, 1979).

12. Michael Anderson, "The Impact upon Family Relationships on the Elderly of Changes since Victorian Times in Governmental Income-Maintenance Provision," in *Family, Bureaucracy and the Elderly*, ed. Ethel Shanas and Marvin Sussman (Durham, N.C.: Duke University Press, 1977).

13. Jan Stehouwer, "Relations between Generations and the Three Generation Household in Denmark," in *Social Structure and the Family*, ed. Shanas and Strieb.

14. Ethel Shanas, "The Family as a Social Support System in Old Age," *Gerontologist* 19, no. 2 (1979): 169–174.

15. Robert Atchley, *The Social Forces of Later Life* (Belmont, Calif.: Wadsworth Publishing Co., 1972).

16. Charles Mindel, "Multigenerational Family Households: Recent Trends and Implications for the Future," *Gerontologist* 19, no. 5 (1979): 456–463.

17. Eugene Litwak, "Extended Kin Relations in an Industrial Democratic Society," in *Social Structure and the Family*, ed. Shanas and Strieb.

18. William Quinn and George Hughston, "The Family as a Natural Support System for the Aged," mimeographed (Blacksburg, Va.: Virginia Polytechnic Institute and State University, 1979).

19. Carla Masciocchi, Walter Poulshock, and Stanley Brody, "Impairment Levels of Ill Elderly: Institutional and Community Perspectives," mimeographed (Philadelphia: University of Pennsylvania, 1979).

20. Johnathan York and Robert Calsyn, "Family Involvement in Nursing Homes," *Gerontologist* 17, no. 6 (1979): 501-505.

21. Ibid.

22. Ethel Shanas and Philip Hauser, "Zero Population Growth and the Family Life of Old People," *Journal of Social Issues* 30, no. 4 (1974): 79-92.

23. See Stanley Brody, Walter Poulshock, and Carla Masciocchi, "The Family Caring Unit: A Major Consideration in the Long-Term Support System," *Gerontologist* 18, no. 6 (1978): 556-561; Marvin Sussman, Donna Vanderwyst, and Gwendolyn Williams, "Will You Still Need Me, Will You Still Feed Me When I'm 64," mimeographed (Winston-Salem, N.C.: Wake Forest University, 1976); Litwak, "Extended Kin Relations," pp. 290-326; and Marvin Sussman, "Incentives and Family Environments for the Elderly," mimeographed (Cleveland: Case Western Reserve, 1976).

24. Marvin Sussman, "Relationships of Adult Children to Their Parents in the United States," in *Social Structure and the Family*, ed. Shanas and Strieb.

25. Shanas, "Family as a Social Support System," pp. 169-174.

26. Ibid; Masciocchi, Poulshock, and Brody, "Impairment Levels."

27. Brody, Poulshock, and Masciocchi, "Family Caring Unit," pp. 556-561.

28. James Callahan, Lawrence Diamond, Janet Giele and Robert Morris, "Responsibility of the Family for Their Severely Disabled Elders," *Health Care Financing Review* 1, no. 3 (1978): 29-48.

29. Brody, Poulshock, and Masciocchi, "Family Caring Unit," George Maddox, "Families as Context and Resource in Chronic Illness," in *Long Term Care: A Handbook for Researchers, Planners and Providers*, ed. Sylvia Sherwood (New York: Spectrum Publications, 1975).

30. Brody, Poulshock, and Masciocchi, "Family Caring Unit," pp. 556--561.

31. Peter Townsend, "The Effects of Family Structure on the Likelihood of Admission to an Institution in Old Age: The Application of a General Theory," in *Social Structure and the Family: Generational Relations*, ed. Ethel Shanas and Gordon Strieb (Englewood Cliffs, N.J.: Prentice-Hall, 1965) pp. 163-178.

32. Shanas, "Family as a Social Support System," pp. 169-174.

33. Masciocchi, Poulshock, and Brody, "Impairment Levels."

34. Callahan, Diamond, Giele, and Morris, "Responsibility," pp. 29-48.

35. Ibid.

36. Townsend, "Effects of Family Structure," pp. 163-178.

37. Alvin Schorr, ". . . Thy Father and Thy Mother . . .' a Second Look at Filial Responsibility and Family Policy" (Washington, D.C.: Department of Health and Human Services, Social Security Administration, no. 13-11953, July 1980).

38. William Fullerton, "Finding Money and Paying for Long-Term Care Services—The Devil's Briarpatch," mimeographed (Silver Spring, Md.: Fullerton, Jones and Wolkstein—Health Policy Alternatives, Inc., 1980).

39. Merlin Taber, Steve Anderson, and C. Jean Rogers, "Implementing Community Care in Illinois: Issues of Cost and Targeting in a Statewide Program," *Gerontologist* 20, no. 3 (1980).

40. Anderson, "Impact upon Family Relationships."

2

The Family Support Program

As the United States moves gradually toward a home-care entitlement for the chronically disabled, the government's stance in relation to the family appears inconsistent and ambivalent. The Family Support Program (FSP) was undertaken for the purpose of exploring and anticipating the policy issues in a two-tier entitlement strategy. In such a plan, the disabled elderly without families receive the most help, with the public assuming full responsibility for maintaining them at home. For those with family resources, publicly financed services would be offered through such programs as FSP only to complement family efforts. Basic caretaking responsibility would remain explicitly with families.

The FSP served disabled elderly and their families from October 1976 through September 1979. Ninety-six families were in service for at least six months, eighty-four for at least one year, and forty-eight for at least two years. At full capacity, the annual program budget reached nearly $300,000.

Assumptions, Objectives, and Questions

The FSP was conceived as a model for the more modest and ancillary public-sector strategy that would complement family care. Services were then conceptualized as incentives to families to sustain their efforts. The goals, design, and analysis focused on incentive strategies and effects that are compatible with public-sector programming. The following assumptions were incorporated in the design (the first four concern the family, and the last three concern public policy):

1. Most adults accept an obligation to provide mutual support throughout the life span of the family.
2. Parents and children are favorably disposed toward one another.
3. Chronically impaired elderly and adult family members are mentally competent and know their own interests.
4. Families' limitations on functional assistance are structural, not attitudinal.
5. Families should be encouraged to provide functional assistance to impaired relatives.
6. Public benefits should support but not replace family effort.

13

7. Incentives should be flexible enough to satisfy diverse family care patterns
    without distorting them and should guarantee equal treatment and benefit
    equity among eligible families.

The following objectives and research questions for FSP were derived
directly from these assumptions:

Short-Range Objectives
1. Recruit families with seriously impaired elderly members.
2. Promptly engage eligible families in service negotiations and agreements.
3. Secure stable service packages and monitor quality of care.

Long-Range Objectives
4. Encourage persistence of family in maintenance efforts.
5. Delay institutionalization.

Research Questions
1. What maintenance functions do families perform for impaired elderly
    members?
2. How does the family organize itself as a service-producing unit? What are
    the constraints on family service?
3. How can the impersonalization and standardization of bureaucratically
    organized services be made compatible with the affective and spontaneous
    attributes of family life?
4. How can the impaired older person's interests be guarded against a family's
    tendency either to reject or overprotect?
5. How do families incorporate service incentives into their life-styles?
6. Do incentives influence a family's willingness or ability to sustain its main-
    tenance efforts?
7. How can an incentive program be integrated with other public benefits for
    the disabled elderly?

From its inception, it was assumed that the FSP would operate for at least
three years. The analytical emphasis, therefore, would be on the short- and
intermediate-range effects that might materialize in that period of time. Of
course, staff members were also interested in discouraging families from placing
their impaired elders in nursing homes. A commonly stated objective for home-
care programs is to delay unnecessary institutionalization. Although this is a
popular and desirable purpose, it has proved extremely difficult to test even with
experimental designs and large programs. It was decided that an intensive analysis of the family, which considered its performance as service provider and its
relationship to formal service organizations, would be a more realistic and a
more useful product. It was believed that the analysis would enable greater

precision and clarity in program designs and measurements of outcomes for long-term care. The data have been organized and presented to elucidate the concept of maintenance as an important social objective and as an alternative to the rehabilitation model for long-term care.

Throughout the analysis, implications are drawn from the FSP experience for the delivery of services in the public sector. The performance of this project, therefore, is implicitly measured by standards applicable to public programs rather than by standards typically exercised in private social agencies. Although the standards are similar in some instances, in many they are not. Experience with uncontrollable expenses and the abuse of public funds for institutional long-term care requires that new home-care models for public entitlements be critically judged by high standards.

Personnel and Administration

The Community Service Society of New York (CSS) conducted the project and funded it from its own resources.

The size of the staff varied slightly throughout the life of the project. There was a period of small expansion, routine turnover, and then reduction as the project reached termination. The core staff essentially consisted of a director (half-time), a program coordinator, a casework supervisor (half-time), two full-time caseworkers, one assistant caseworker, and three homemakers. The homemaker staff was expanded with CETA (Comprehensive Employment and Training Act) workers later in the program, and substantial sums were spent on the purchase of home care from vendor agencies throughout the program. Two social-work students were assigned to the program each year.

The administrative style of a program can be described in terms of the degree of structural complexity, centralized authority, procedural discipline, and predetermined decision criteria. Prior to the initiation of FSP, this same service staff had functioned as a casework unit within the agency, providing counseling, advocacy, and some homemaker services to the elderly. The administrative style in FSP primarily reflected the traditional professional culture of the office.

For a small office, the structure was fairly complex. (See figure 2-1.) The authority was centralized. Although case supervision and program administration were structurally separated, the administrator was also an active supervisor who participated in decision making concerning most cases. Determination of eligibility, benefit level, and services provided resembled a case-assessment model in some respects. The variables associated with these decisions were neither highly standardized nor specified in advance. Flexibility in assessment was more compatible with the philosophy of the office than was standardized assessment. In summary, operational control and consistency were centralized since they depended upon the personal judgments of the administrator.

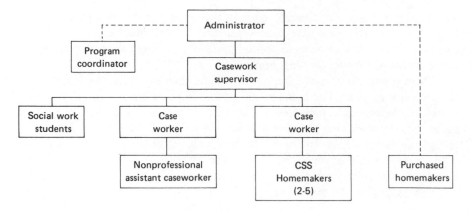

Figure 2–1. Family Support Program Organizational Chart

Eligibility Standards and Clientele Characteristics

With an analytical commitment to the study of families and disability, FSP established the family as the basic unit of eligibility. To be eligible, families were required to have at least one functionally impaired elderly member and at least one supporting member. A supporting member could be a spouse, a sibling, a child, or another relative, as long as there was an observable demarcation between needing service and rendering service.

A serious and chronic level of impairment was required.[1] Impairment was defined as an inability to maintain one's self independently in the community. Project staff hoped to serve a sample of families with a continuum of maintenance needs, excluding the extremes. The project did not have the resources to purchase around-the-clock care; nonetheless some families were admitted when a combination of family, public-sector, and FSP resources equaled such care. At the other extreme, the project attempted to reject families where declining performance rather than serious impairment characterized the condition of the older person. Program guidelines stipulated that there must be "evidence that the elderly member is unable to perform [some] essential daily functions because of one, or a combination of the following disabilities: bowel and bladder, vision, hearing, speech, mobility, transfer, hand and arm movement, or confusion." Serving mildly impaired elderly was discouraged since public policy in the United States is formulated in response to categorical need. Also the elderly with slight impairment are less likely to require routine services. The plausibility of agency intervention depends to some extent upon the efficiency obtainable with standard procedures and routines.

The staff did not employ a standardized instrument for measuring impairment during the admission process, but impairment was measured subsequently in research interviews. Physical and mental functioning was assessed by using the Functioning for Independent Living scale (see Appendix A), which rates the older person's ability to perform the tasks of everyday life: vision, hearing and speech, mobility, transfer, hand and arm movement, and bowel and bladder control. Mental assessment in areas of memory, identity, speech wandering, and nonconventional behavior was also measured.

Functioning for Independent Living (FIL) scores ranged from 0 to 38. The median score for clients was 10.1, and the average score was 12.3. The disability scores were concentrated in the lower portion of the range (table 2-1). A more complete description of disability and the instrument appears in the Appendix.

The following case illustrations will provide a better qualitative impression of the experience with disabilities reflected in the FIL scores. (The following brief descriptive accounts are preceded by the FIL scale scores: V = vision, HS = hearing and speech, M = mobility, T = transfer, HA = hand and arm movement, BB = bowel and bladder, and Conf = confusion.) The first two accounts belong to category I; scores range from zero to five, with the impairment level being mild.[a]

V	HS	M	T	HA	BB	Conf.
0	0	0	2	0	0	0

Mrs. Crane assured me that while her sister complains a lot, she remains quite self-sufficient. She dresses herself, toilets herself, and takes care of all her personal needs including giving herself insulin injections. Ms. B said she goes to see her sister approximately every other week, usually on weekends because she works full-time.

"She can manage herself pretty well with the help the homemaker gives. She puts on a big act. When anyone else asks, everything is fine. When it comes to me, everything is wrong. . . . The doctor said he didn't feel she had to be in a nursing home and if she could get a homemaker and stay in her own home, she'd be happier." [Score = 2]

Table 2-1
Distribution of Functional Impairment Scores at Time of Entry

Categorical Levels	Percent
Low (0–5)	26
Moderate (6–11)	27
Serious (12–17)	19
Severe (18–25)	20
Very severe (26 +)	8

[a]All of the names used in case studies are fictitious.

V	HS	M	T	HA	BB	Conf.
2	0	1	0	0	1	0

Mrs. Stein wears bifocals and says she cannot read fine print. She has difficulty hearing at times, but she can hear well enough to permit essential conversation even if the speaker's voice is only slightly raised. She does not wear a mechanical device. She can walk up to eight blocks and climb stairs with assistance. She is generally active and goes out often to eat, or to the senior citizens' center.

"She suffers from weakness; gets headaches and gets dizzy. . . ." Her vision and hearing are also affected, "but not to the point that it's a crisis . . . that's why I wanted minimal amount of time of homemaker service." [Score = 4]

The next two cases are from category II; scores are between six and eleven and represent a moderate amount of impairment:

V	HS	M	T	HA	BB	Conf.
0	0	6	0	2	0	0

"Her vision is not bad; she has always had a disability in her left eye. Her hearing is fine, but her speech is somewhat garbled since her stroke . . . but we can still have adequate conversation. Now as for her mobility, I'd say since her stroke she is not able to maintain her balance. She's unable to overcome this physiologically. In addition, she has a fear of falling. That's why we needed someone to walk her.

"We saw that she needed someone as a companion, someone to take her for walks and help her get out. She felt boxed in and it was very depressing. . . . Well, I call regularly, invite her to family get-togethers, religious celebrations, the theater. I don't do her household chores. After her stroke, I took her to all the doctors and treatments. Since then she's been trying to do it on her own and just needed a little bit of help." [Score = 8]

V	HS	M	T	HA	BB	Conf.
0	2	1	1	2	2	3

"Mr. Gunther has suffered from Parkinson's disease since 1961. He stands stooped to a right angle and cannot speak intelligently or loudly. . . . His memory functions are deteriorating. He often thinks it's Sabbath, and dresses to go to the synagogue. . . . He has walked to the synagogue but often cannot maintain himself in a standing position for long without falling. He can perform most transfers independently except for getting in and out of an automobile.

"He walks stooped. Everybody looks. He walks into a pole. He don't see. He don't look up. . . . I couldn't stand someone here twenty-four hours a day anyway. . . . Yes, I leave him alone, usually in the afternoons since he sleeps for two hours after lunch. But many times when I come back, he's fallen. . . . I feed him at supper and then he'll fall asleep. Sometimes as long as two hours on the clock. I get so excited that I scream at him at the top of my lungs." [Score = 11]

The following case is from category III; scores are between twelve and seventeen and represent a serious level of impairment:

V	HS	M	T	HA	BB	Conf.
0	4	4	2	4	0	0

Mrs. Marquez, who is very weak, has asthma, emphysema, and walks with a walker. She is apparently unsteady on her feet and had to have a pin put in her hip as she has fallen a couple of times. Mrs. M. has an additional disability—she is deaf. . . . She is able to eat by herself, but needs help dressing and bathing.

"Everything has to be written down. . . . The problem is trying to get meaningful thoughts or conversation down on paper. . . . I told Mrs. R. [social worker], that we're trying to hold off sending mother to a nursing home as long as possible. I asked if we could have a nurse to come in for two days. . . . I tried bathing her once, and I'm sure I did it all wrong. I'm sure I didn't hold her right—she was like a rag doll. I'm really terrified to handle her now." [Score = 14]

The following two cases are from category IV; scores are between eighteen and twenty-five and represent a severe level of impairment:

V	HS	M	T	HA	BB	Conf.
0	2	6	6	6	1	1

"I have to get Mama up, dress her, and bathe her. She eats by herself, but everything else I have to do for her. She could really go out more than she does, but she has spasms, and she's afraid she'll have one in church or on the street with other people around. She has spasms every week or so, and I have to be here. I can't just go in back and leave her alone. She has to have somebody around all the time." [Score = 22]

V	HS	M	T	HA	BB	Conf.
2	2	1	6	2	0	11

Mr. Bell is reported to have hardening of the arteries, and the beginnings of Parkinson's disease. His legs are affected and so he walks very slowly. He requires full-time care and cannot be left alone for a period of time. Once when he was left alone, he was found in the hallway without shoes and socks, speaking in Spanish.

"If I say, 'Open your mouth and take your dentures out,' he will put his hand in my mouth, or try to pull the faucet or soap dish off the wall. . . . Every night it's the same thing. I get a little nervous [about it]. It's a little exasperating." [Score = 24]

These final two cases are from category V; scores are from twenty-six and over and represent very severe impairment:

V	HS	M	T	HA	BB	Conf.
0	2	6	5	6	3	6

"His vision is good with glasses. He watches TV. He can pick out a few words from the newspaper and can read his own name when he sees it. But his whole right side is affected due to a stroke. His speech—he can't convey what he's trying to say. He has automatic speech—he repeats his name. We have a speech therapist come in once a week. He can't walk at all; his knees are constricted. If he could use his right hand at all, he might be able to use the walker, but he can't. I do exercises with him but they don't seem to work. He can't get out of bed or any of those other things. He needs to be lifted. He can't walk. He can't lift anything at all. He wets himself a lot. He's not incontinent, but yet he does have frequent urinary and bladder accidents. His memory is fair, but it's hard to say; he can't really talk so I can't say. He does need to be reminded to take his medicine or do his exercises, though. No, he can't always remember his name or address; it's because of the aphasia. Well, because of the stroke, he can't speak coherently."

"I help him with his speech therapy; I put the straps on his legs and wrist so they can take his EKG over the phone. I wash him, shave him, comb his hair, wash his feet; I help with the physical therapy. I have to wipe him after the toilet. I have to do all the household chores, all the cooking. I have to take him to the pot. It seems like I give up all my time. I'm on call round-the-clock." [Score = 28]

V	HS	M	T	HA	BB	Conf.
4	0	6	6	6	6	10

"Well, she has cataracts and can't read anything anymore. No, not labels, but she can still see some. Her hearing and speech, they're okay. They're the only things that still are okay. She can't walk no more. She's using a wheelchair when I can get her into it. No, she can't move by herself. I gots to help her out of bed, and everywhere. She's too weak to lift anything, I mean anything. She's got no strength not even to stay sitting up. Oh, does she have accidents! She's incontinent. . . . She's senile. She can't remember nothing, not her name, and she has no idea where she's living. She babbles incoherently. I don't understand her. She can't wander, no way, but she would if she could. Oh, she'll tear off her clothes sometimes, just throw them on the floor. I don't know where she gets the strength. Sometimes I have to sedate her, but I don't like to do that." [Score = 38]

Relying primarily on informal agency networks, FSP received approximately 450 service inquiries in three years. Most of those declared ineligible were rejected on the basis of such criteria as residence outside the service area or incomes well above the specified limit. Assessment of serious impairment did not play as large a role in identifying ineligibles as originally intended. A substantial proportion of client families (26 percent) ultimately came from the lowest disability category (table 2-1). Denying service to applicants is a troublesome matter for most staff, particularly in private agencies that have a historical self-perception of benevolence and compassion. Any public program would need to rely more heavily on structured disability testing for eligibility purposes.

The program design called for the staff to screen out families that could not assume primary responsibility. Some applicants were rejected when the staff suspected a need for protective services or suspected incompetence among family members. When these criteria were invoked, the reasons appeared complicated and obscure. Problems in standardizing such criteria are explored in chapter 6.

Because of the small nonprobability sample in this demonstration, selectivity in admission was not an onerous problem. In a public-entitlement program, however, such decisions inevitably would be controversial. To avoid such controversy, standards for testing family incompetence would need to be very high and very explicit. Even the most rigorous procedures for estimating incompetence have not proven highly reliable.

In slightly fewer than half of the cases, applications were made in response to an abrupt deterioration in the condition of the older person (25 percent), a change in the family (14 percent), or a change in formal home-care services (10 percent). In the last category, the problem typically was the expiration of Medicare financing for services of home health aides. There was no immediate crisis in the remaining cases.

The average age of the disabled elderly in the FSP program was 77 years. Over three-fourths (77 percent) of the elderly were female, and 23 percent were male. Fifty-five percent of the elderly were white, 40 percent were black, and 3 percent were Hispanic. Only 22 percent of the elderly had family incomes over $6,000 per year, and in over 50 percent of the cases, family income was less than $4,000 per year. Seventeen percent were receiving SSI. Most (90 percent) were receiving social security, and 39 percent had private pensions in addition to social security. Approximately one-third lived alone, one-third with a spouse, and one-third with other relatives. (See table 2-2.)

Approximately three-quarters of the families were referred to the FSP through informal private-agency networks. Early in the program, a feature article in a major city paper produced approximately one hundred inquiries. This brought some families into the program who were not previously in a service network. The effect of publicity on applications suggests that it is a very promising recruitment strategy. Small programs such as FSP that lack the resources to satisfy the possible demand for assistance, however, are reluctant to advertise widely. Nonetheless such reservation should not be necessary in an entitlement program. In fact, it would be desirable to test the response rate to a widely advertised home-care program in a larger demonstration.

Table 2–2
Case Family Characteristics (N = 96)

Source of referral	
Social agencies	26%
FSP clients	23
Response to advertisement	20
Other CSS clients	17
Hospitals	6
Living arrangements of disabled elderly	
Lived alone	35
Shared household with relative other than spouse	33
Shared household with spouse	32
Income of disabled elderly	
Under $4,000	57
$4,000–5,999	20
$6,000–7,999	18
$8,000–9,999	5
Marital status of disabled elderly	
Married	33
Widowed	63
Other	4
Ethnicity of disabled elderly	
Black	39
White	55
Other	6
Sex of primary family support	
Male	25
Female	75
Relationship of primary family support to disabled member	
Adult children	63
Son	16
Daughter	47
Spouse	24
Sister	8
Employment of primary family support	
Employed	52
Unemployed	14
Retired	26
Housewife	6
Other	2

In 63 percent of the cases, the family member with primary responsibility was a son or daughter, and usually (47 percent) it was the daughter. The average age among this group was fifty-two. Sixty-five percent of these family members were also employed. Half of the adult children with primary responsibility were single (48 percent) or widowed (8 percent). Two-thirds shared an apartment or lived within walking distance of the impaired older person.

The second major group with primary responsibility for care was spouses (24 percent). Husbands and wives appeared in supporting roles in approximately equal proportions. The average age of husbands was seventy-eight; wives were considerably younger (average age sixty-nine). Only two spouses were employed.

In the remaining families (13 percent) no one person was clearly identified with primary responsibility. Supportive efforts were divided among a cohort of secondary family sources that provided more-casual care at irregular intervals. These secondary sources averaged fifty years of age. Most (79 percent) were self-employed. Men and women assumed this role in equal proportions.

Procedures

The planning of the demonstration called for clearly demarcated stages of application, admission, service, and termination, but these distinctions were not always sustained. The service staff preferred greater flexibility in determining eligibility and service response. Discrepancies between the intended procedures (as described here) and their application are described in chapter 6.

All telephone applications were screened by the service staff director and casework supervisor. They also assigned staff to the cases, made the final eligibility decision, and approved all provisional service plans made by the staff and families. This hierarchical arrangement offers the promise of greater internal consistency when criteria for eligibility and service are not defined. Even when the authority is centralized, some inconsistency is inevitable, however.

The original plan called for the staff to proceed with a family meeting once eligibility had been determined. Staff members conducted family meetings at a time and location convenient for the family. Nearly all such meetings were held outside the agency office. Ultimately the staff reserved eligibility decisions until after the family meeting, preferring an opportunity to examine the functioning and "competence" of the family unit more closely before committing resources.

The family meeting was the crucial component in early case handling. Project success rested on the ability to convene meetings quickly, obtain family attendance, and define a service package. Staff members were successful at scheduling and conducting meetings. Families did not object to the idea and generally seemed to appreciate the opportunity to air their grievances. They came with the expectation of improving their situation.

Program protocol called for the practitioner to reiterate program objectives and strategy, review existing family maintenance supports, solicit requests for the extent and nature of the agency's participation, and commit agency resources in response to stated requests. The family also received a program brochure that suggested possible services such as homemaker and personal care, assistance with public entitlements, transportation, and weekend relief. The program description given to families was to have emphasized the leading role expected of family members in defining services. The staff member was expected to solicit requests and respond to them. The challenge was to match the families' maintenance experience with the practitioners' knowledge of entitlements and service-delivery mechanisms, plus their broader experience with solutions to recurring problems. The goal was to intervene as little as possible in the actual decision making (service definition) while providing the information (counseling) necessary for the family to make an intelligent, well-informed decision.

Further complications were expected when families were uncertain about what they wanted or did not clearly articulate their needs. Experienced practitioners also needed to be cautious of carrying preconceived notions into the family meeting and filtering or biasing the family's expression of maintenance problems. The importance and complexity of the task placed a heavy responsibility on the practitioner's management of the meeting. Discussions with families began by the worker explaining, "We have a wide variety of services to offer." From this introduction, the worker was expected to assist the family in forming and expressing its preferences.

In every case, the worker prepared a written mutual agreement, a statement that included a brief summary of what the family provided and would continue to provide and the FSP service commitments. This agreement formally asserted that continued participation of the family was a condition of continued receipt of services.

The caseworkers were responsible for monitoring. The format and frequency were not specified in advance. It was anticipated that relatively small case loads (approximately twenty-five per worker), combined with supervision of homemakers and contact through counseling, would achieve formal monitoring purposes indirectly.

Domain of Service

The project offered homemakers, case management, entitlement advocacy, and financial assistance for the purchase of basic amenities. FSP had the advantage of operating a broader service domain than is typical of categorical public programs, and it also had greater control over resources. The agency provided the staff with approximately $100,000 per year for the purchase of direct services, so service arrangements could be made promptly. The use of CSS funds created an opportunity to finance care for those with incomes above the Medicaid eligibility limits. Service arrangements could also be organized quickly for those who subsequently obtained a homemaker through Medicaid. For the FSP clients, delays typically associated with Medicaid application were not obstacles to the initiation of service. In this respect, the FSP staff role went beyond the means available in the typical case-management program. The importance of this feature should not be underestimated; the availability of a prompt and reliable home-care alternative is a decisive factor in planning the care of hospitalized and severely impaired elderly. FSP's unique resources gave it significance as a demonstration that is not duplicated in other case-management programs now underway. The principal sources of service were the professional staff, the homemakers, homemaker services purchased with CSS funds from other agencies, and homemakers financed by Medicaid.

Budget

At full capacity, the budget for the FSP was nearly $300,000 on an annualized basis (table 2-3). Professional staff and associated indirect costs essentially were constant throughout the program, and changes primarily reflected annual salary increments.[2] The planned allocation of dollars for the purchase of home care rose dramatically from $15,000 for the first year to approximately $130,000 annually during the second year as the number of cases expanded.

After the first year, approximately eighty to ninety families were enrolled in the program at any one time. With total expenditures between $240,000 and $290,000, the average annual expenditures per client varied between $2,800 and $3,400. On a monthly basis, expenditures varied between $233 and $283 per client.[3]

Overall budget figures can be divided further into management and direct-service expenses (table 2-3). Direct service includes homemakers purchased with CSS funds, homemakers directly employed by CSS, and financial assistance for other purposes, such as vacation, recreation, transportation, household equipment and maintenance, and other miscellaneous items. Management costs include professionals' salaries[4] and fringe benefits, and other indirect office expenses (table 2-4).

Table 2-3
Annualized FSP Expenditure Estimates

Costs	At Month 12	At Month 24
Administrative and case-management	$138,100	$149,000
Direct service	99,900	143,625
Total	238,000	292,625
Administrative and case-management costs as a percent of total	58	51

Note: Expenditures in months 12 and 24 are multiplied by 12 to obtain an annualized estimate of the program in two phases. These estimates indicate the range of administrative to direct-service-cost ratios that can be expected at near-optimal and optimal performance.

Table 2–4
Administrative and Case-Management Costs

Items	Expenditures
Salaries	
Professional[a]	$ 80,600
Clerical and other support staff	25,300
Total	105,900
Indirect	
General office service	10,200
Data processing	4,000
Process shop and stenographic services	3,400
Total	17,600
Other	
Staff expenses	2,250
Telephone	3,000
Rent	7,280
Miscellaneous	2,070
Total	14,600
Total	$138,100

Note: Annual average costs estimated from budget for quarter of the fiscal year 1978–1979, July through September.

[a]The staff members were a half-time director, three caseworkers with master of socialwork degrees, and one geriatric assistant.

The cost ratio of management to direct service is one measure of efficiency in administration. In the FSP, management costs ranged from 51 to 59 percent of total expenditures. Although there is no existing cost-ratio standard for measuring administrative efficiency, administrative cost rates of this magnitude may be typical of private agencies and small home-care projects.[5] For a public entitlement program, however, they would be burdensome. Obviously administrative costs in varying program formats should be given close attention in future demonstrations. The degree of professionalization and frequency of monitoring are the major cost variables.

A closer examination of direct-service expenditures provides one indicator of diversity in purchases. As table 2–5 indicates, approximately 90 percent of all direct-service expenditures went for the purchase of homemaker services. The staff accepted the principle of offering clients a wide variety of services, but it appears that a traditional homemaker service was generally the result of this strategy. Approximately 1 percent of the direct-service budget went for the purchase of household equipment, home maintenance, and other miscellaneous items. It is essential to recognize that the distinguishing feature of the program rests on its ability to command resources for the purchase of care, and the nature and format of service delivery is not itself substantially modified.

Table 2–5
Time Samples of Direct-Service Expenditures

Expenditure Items for One Month	Time Intervals			
	Year = 1	Year = 1.5	Year = 2	Year = 2.5
Total amount of homemaker services	$7,600	$10,936	$10,329	$6,228
Purchased homemaker	6,200	7,886	6,769	4,228
CSS homemaker	1,400	3,040	3,560	2,000
Vacation/recreation	225	697	1,063	732
Transportation	160	222	146	54
Household equipment and maintenance, and miscellaneous	230	114	84	160
Total	$8,215	$11,969	$11,622	$7,174
All homemaker services as percent of total direct service expenditure	92%	91%	89%	87%
Number of clients and average expenditure	Data not available	$N = 67$ $\overline{X} = \$179$	$N = 66$ $\overline{X} = \$176$	$N = 47$ $\overline{X} = \$153$

Terminations

Thirty-seven cases were terminated during the data-collection period, after at least six months of service. Thirteen terminations (35 percent) were attributable to nursing-home placement (see table 2–6). The figures in the table underestimate the termination rate by death, since a sample survey of thirteen terminations drawn from the thirty-seven cases revealed that some survived for only a brief period in nursing homes.

In the sample of thirteen terminated cases, eleven were terminated for reasons of dramatic deterioration in the condition of the disabled person. In the remaining two cases, either the client moved away or the family obtained the desired level of homemaker service through Medicaid and preferred no further contact with the program.

Among these eleven cases, there was a general pattern of very high disability. With one exception, these clients were in the highest disability category at time of termination. The following excerpt from a case is typical:

> Mrs. Wolfe deteriorated further and had several accidents. She fell on the corner of a table, had a black eye, and received six stitches. Later she fell out of bed, had three broken ribs, and a concussion. After two weeks in the hospital, she went directly to a nursing home.

Five of these eleven clients died with a few weeks of termination. One of the five clients died at home, and the remainder died in hospitals or nursing homes after

Table 2–6
Reasons for Termination

Reason	End of First Year	End of Second Year[a]
Entered nursing home	2	10
Death	4	9
Moved out of area	3	4
Family withdrew or was defined by staff as uncooperative	3	2
Total	12	25

[a]Frequencies are noncumulative.

a few weeks. In every case, the process of nursing-home placement followed brief hospitalization. It appears that hospitalization occurred in response to illness or injury rather than as a preplanned route to nursing home placement. Hospital physicians and social workers who generally favored nursing-home placement at discharge, were very influential:

> The [doctor at the] hospital said there's no way she could make it. We wanted to take her back and they said her coming back really wouldn't work out.

> The doctor told me it was "high time" she was in a nursing home.

> We took her to the hospital after the fall. There were no broken bones but the doctor said she needed round-the-clock care. After the fall, it was out of our hands.

The presence of incontinence, confusion, and assaultive behavior were accepted by hospital professionals as indicators of necessary institutional care. With one exception, every family expressed a strong desire to bring its elderly member home from the hospital rather than to proceed with placement. The one exception involved a confused and physically assaultive man who had hit his daughter several times.

Families agreed on placements when they became convinced that the obstacles to further home care were insurmountable. Family members gave the impression they were not just persistent but tenacious in their commitment to home care. Even in the Wolfe case, the daughter was very reluctant to have her mother placed in a nursing home, according to the case record: "I cried for months. Now I've concluded it was the best move. But I would still bring her home if I had a full-time attendant." Other families expressed their reluctance over placement. One family member said, "If I had longer homemaker hours, twenty-four hours a day, I'd have her with me now" and another expressed the same thought: "It was traumatic for both of us. I was worried all the time." But then she added, "Now it's a great load off my husband's mind. We have a more stable home life."

This close examination of terminations indicates that services were strong incentives for families to resist nursing-home placement. Within the design of the demonstration, this is the best available evidence. Given the FSP admission practices, there is undoubtedly an interaction effect between selection and treatment. Whether the incentives caused persistence or enabled already-persistent families to persevere is moot. It is more important to note the percentage of families that continued with home care until the death of the disabled person, the reluctance for placement even with states of extreme disability, and the number of family members who cited homemaker and service limitations as the central obstacle to continued care at home.[6]

Notes

1. Other eligibility criteria reflected practical constraints rather than policy considerations. They were local residence of the impaired person within one hour's commuting time, annual gross income of the impaired person less than $8,000, and consent of the family to participate in research.

2. The original staff was expanded by the addition of one worker who assumed responsibilities for some FSP clients but also worked in other areas of the agency. Ultimately her FSP role diminished, so costs attributable to her have not been figured in these calculations. It can be assumed, therefore, that the professional staff budget is slightly underestimated.

3. Average program expenditure figure is not a measure of total services received. All families had varying levels of family support, and many had Medicaid-financed homemakers.

4. At some point the line between direct service and case management is blurred. In some instances, professional social workers were involved in counseling independent of case-monitoring activities. Typically, however, these tasks were combined in one activity. Also some expenses treated as direct service were administrative. A portion of $70,000 to $90,000 allocated to the purchases of homemaker care is, of course, attributable to administrative costs in the homemaker agencies.

5. The cost ratio does not appear to be out of line with other, similar programs. In chapter 7, administrative cost comparisons are made with other case-management and homemaker projects on which published cost data are available.

6. For similar results see Marvin Sussman, "Social and Economic Supports and Family Environments for the Elderly," mimeographed (Winston-Salem, N.C.: Lake Forest University, 1979).

3

Flexibility and Constraints in Family Care

As providers of care, families are highly decentralized, and their functions have little public exposure. The actual tasks they perform to maintain impaired elderly members are not well documented. Because of their experience and responsibility, they offer a very knowledgeable account of the necessities of home care. This chapter presents a detailed, descriptive analysis of their activities and constraints. It reconstructs patterns of family maintenance, and draws similarities and distinctions between family and present organizational patterns of service delivery. Motivations, resources, and constraints that lie behind the family patterns are examined also because knowledge of the criteria by which a family perceives and measures its own capacity to care should influence future policy decisions regarding the extent of family responsibility for care.

Diversity and Flexibility

The level of care provided by any one family could be exceptionally high:

> I prepare the food for the week. She may remember to heat it on a hot plate, or I call her and remind her to eat. Sometimes she wants breakfast at 7:00 p.m. because she'd gone to bed at 4:00 p.m. She thought it was a new day, so I call her several times and keep her in touch—tell her the time and the like. I do her ironing, wash, her shopping. I take her to the store and let her pick out what she wants. She feels she's still able to do things this way. I do her heavy cleaning. I go up every night for four or five hours. That's hard on my husband. He's not used to it. My sister does much of this work too. She bathes her, gives her the personal care like washing and setting her hair. I take her down to my house for dinner. We try to take her out on weekends when we can. We help her out financially. We pay the rent.

> We used to have mother take a shower in the morning before we went to work, but we discovered that there wasn't enough time and things were too rushed, so now we do this in the evening. In the morning, Robert fixes mother's breakfast. Then we have her get dressed. If there's no time for that, Sadie [the homemaker] dresses her. In the evening we ask her if she ate, fix her dinner, help her undress, help her take her shower. I watch her to make sure she brushes her teeth and puts on deodorant. When we go away overnight, we usually take mother with us unless it is an imposition on the people we are visiting.

If we have to go away overnight and can't take her with us, we get
someone to stay over with her, and it usually costs about $15 a day.

Sixteen categories of family support activities are displayed in table 3–1,
along with the frequency distributions for each category. Many of the distributions are bimodal, with respondents concentrated at the upper and lower ends
of the distributions. This apparently reflects the wide variation in disability
among the service recipients. The services most frequently provided by family
members are preparing meals, light housecleaning, administering or supervising
medication, and assisting or supervising grooming and personal hygiene. The
most infrequently provided services are heavy-duty housecleaning, making home
repairs, assisting with transfer, assisting with transportation, and supplementing
constant supervision of the disabled person.

In performing personal care functions, family attentiveness to individual
needs, routines, wishes, and even whims of the older person is obvious:

We get her up and we put her on the loveseat in the living room and
feed her. We keep her up for two to three hours and put her back to
bed. About every two weeks or so we wash her hair, give her a blue
rinse, put lipstick on her and put her hair in a french twist with floral
combs. She looks nice and she likes it.

My sister also massages her hands and legs; takes care of a bed sore;
places pillows between her knees to reduce abrasion and uses heat to
increase warmth since sometimes the water mattress is too cold.

Personal care tended to be brief and episodic. Bathing and grooming an older
person can require perhaps an hour or so early in the morning or late in the
evening. Many of the personal care activities, such as bathing and toileting, were
personally difficult for family members to provide.

We need someone to bathe and wash her down. She can't wash herself
thoroughly at the sink. I can partially help, but she cleans her private
areas herself.

She breaks my rest at night. She gets up maybe two or three times
to go to the bathroom. I put paper on the floor 'cause she doesn't
always make it. But the noise of the paper always wakes me up.

Performance of simple errands such as food shopping shows similar flexibility and tolerance of idiosyncratic preference. For example, many of the
elderly family members were particular about the prices they paid for food.
They would require a family member to bypass the closest small grocery store in
order to take advantage of supermarket bargains. As one family member said,
"I couldn't ask anyone else to do the shopping because I cut out the coupons

from the paper. I go to one store for one thing, and another store for something else, so we can save a couple of dollars." A family member would take the impaired older person shopping if it offered the possibility of exercise and self-expression to the elderly member. Convenience and efficiency were not the principal objectives.

Housekeeping, dusting, vacuuming, marketing, and doing laundry and simple neighborhood errands were readily incorporated into the supporting members' life-style. Family members could accomplish many services, such as laundry and shopping, while doing their own.

Routine home-maintenance tasks, heavy chores, and housekeeping service were also provided by families, although most of the disabled elderly lived in apartments where superintendents assumed some responsibility for home repair. The distinction that home-care organizations make between light and heavy housecleaning does not appear among family members; these were merely additional housecleaning tasks that had to be done. Family members did a variety of tasks: painting, fixing small appliances, washing windows, even changing light bulbs.

Continuous or nighttime supervision of an impaired person was one of the most difficult services for families to provide. Sometimes the elderly person wandered through the house at night or did not know the difference between day and night and so constantly disrupted the household. The supervision also made it difficult for the family member to go out at night socially.

Families occasionally could rely on a cooperative neighbor to provide simple supervision:

> I go to school every day. I leave early, so before I leave I send my father over to Marion's. She lives right nearby. When he leaves I give two rings on the phone to Marion to let her know he's coming. There's one problem—when he rings the bell and Marion rings him in, he doesn't know what to do. So she has to come down and let him in. He rings the wrong bell a lot and the neighbor on the second floor will come down and let him in.

Families provided some crucial services that home-care organizations do not, such as relocation. The elderly who were trapped in deteriorated neighborhoods often expressed dissatisfaction with their present residences, so adult children sometimes moved a parent closer to them—either into the same building or the same apartment. The purpose usually was to achieve greater security or to facilitate more-intensive care.

Financial management is another routine family service that home-care agencies are reluctant to provide. Agencies rarely seek conservatorships because of the time and monetary costs of obtaining legal authority.

> I have a joint checking account with Mama. She signs checks and I deposit them, so she knows where it goes. Money represents security

Table 3-1
Distribution of Family Activities

Items	At Least Once a Day	Three or Four Times a Week	One or Two Times a Week	One to Three Times a Month	Less than Once a Month	Never or Not Applicable
Shop for personal items and food	15%	20%	35%	15%	5%	10%
Prepare meals	4	14	12	3	7	24
Do light housecleaning (for example, dust, wash dishes, or take out trash)	28	11	18	10	7	26
Do heavy housecleaning (for example, scrub floors, wash windows, or move furniture)	4	1	14	12	15	54
Arrange for or make home repairs (for example, heating, plumbing, painting)	4	0	6	15	25	50
Administer or supervise medication	41	3	4	1	8	43
Sometimes contribute money for expenses	15	4	3	34	10	34
Help with laundry	8	7	26	8	8	43
Supervise or assist with grooming, personal hygiene, or dress (for example, bathing, toileting, clothes selection)	39	3	7	8	5	38
Assist with transfer (for example, moving from bed to chair or from toilet to chair)	27	4	4	4	5	60
Help manage finances (for example, cash social security check, or keep bank account)	11	1	14	45	20	10

Assist in transportation by escorting in a car, taxi, or on public transportation	1	1	8	32	29	29
Assist in physical exercise program (for example, physical therapy or accompanying on walks)	11	7	8	10	3	61
Substitute for the temporarily absent care-giver in order to assure the continual presence of a responsible person	8	1	10	5	12	64
Visit or make social calls (by phone or in person)[a]	28	5	7	4	0	56
Occasionally contribute money for expenses or recreation[a]	3	0	3	9	9	76

[a]Family members who lived with the disabled person were instructed to check the "not applicable" column when answering this question.

to older people. I explain the bank statement to Mama so she knows
where everything goes.

I handle all her finances. That's time-consuming and can be a little
tricky. I pay the bills. She needs drugs that are very expensive. There's
a lot of paperwork in this, and it has to be submitted to Medicaid. I
have to go to the welfare office and have her recertified. That can take
an entire day.

I do her income tax. She handles day-to-day expenses, but if she has
major expenses she always talks to me.

Some family members also made financial contributions to their disabled elderly:
"I give her a little money, but I have to be careful not to jeopardize her eligibility."

Families were found to provide a more diversified mix of services than is
typical of formally organized care. They showed more flexibility in delivery and
more attention to quality than to efficiency. There appears little of the specialization characteristic of formal organizations in the service-delivery style of
families. Within families, light housekeeping, heavy-duty cleaning, and personal
care tasks are performed by the same person. The implicit domain of care
defined by family practice is broader than the present home-care domain.
Family members consider fixing a leaky faucet, installing a prosthetic device,
or shoveling the snow off the sidewalk in winter as legitimate components of
home care for the impaired. Also, family care may be delivered in small units of
time and at awkward hours that preclude the cooperation of efficiency minded
formal organizations. For example, in New York City, homemaker or personal
care generally is not available from agencies in amounts of fewer than three half-
days a week for fewer than four hours at a time.

Restrictions and Conflicts in Family Support

The families served by the FSP generally provided strong support for their
elderly members. All family members, however, operated within specific constraints, and not all family members participated equally.

The most obvious circumstance that can keep some members marginally
involved in care is geographic dispersion. Many family members lived so far from
the older person that direct and extended support was impossible or, at least, a
great inconvenience.

Mr. Goldfarb has two sisters. One lives in New Hampshire. The other
sister in New Jersey tries to visit him on the weekends every four to
eight weeks. It's a long trip. She stays a couple of hours and that's it.
The sister living in New Hampshire does not visit. [Staff]

Family members living in close proximity to the older person might be constrained by employment and other family obligations.

I am working full time, have a house to run, and seeing her everyday took a toll on us.

His [the son's] first shift is from 4 p.m. to 12 a.m. for seven days. He then has a day off. His next schedule is 8 a.m. to 4 p.m. for six days with a day off. He then works from 12 a.m. to 8 p.m. and then has five days off. [Staff]

Children and siblings of disabled members usually had their own families to manage. Adult care givers considered it reasonable to give priority to their own spouse and children. The limitations were more severe when the adult children were working full time and raising young families.

When I asked whether there were other children, both Mrs. G. and Harold, her husband, referred to the son in the Bronx. They were in agreement that he was overwhelmed with his problems of bringing up six children whom he has to "keep after." While they are obviously on good terms, he does not visit often because of his own family responsibilities. [Staff]

Harold Jr. [the primary support] is the youngest of Mrs. Gould's two sons. Harold Jr. has six children, and two are married. One lives in Staten Island and has a variety of health and marital problems of his own and five children whom he is struggling to support. There's a cousin in Brooklyn, but she has problems with her husband. . . . There is another cousin that comes to live with Mrs. Gould. But he only stays when he's having marital problems with his wife. [Staff]

In some instances, the available family members also suffered from debilitating conditions. Many of the principal supporting members were spouses and siblings in their seventies and eighties, and were not expected to contribute vigorously or perform physically demanding tasks.

Personality conflicts and difficult interpersonal relationships also restricted the level of care. Some relatives were reluctant to become involved because of previously strained relations, typically long-standing intergenerational disputes or conflict between the adult children and their spouses. In a few instances the disputes were between the older adult and the spouse.

She does not get along with her son-in-law. He accuses her of being the reason why his wife had to see a psychiatrist. He doesn't pay her rent but gives her about $100 per month and has let her know that he thinks she should have saved more money when she was working. [Staff]

Mrs. Ludlow, who is married and lives with her [disabled] mother, presented the problem of a "personality conflict" between herself and

her mother. Mrs. Ludlow said her mother doesn't like her, and they
have terrible, terrible fights where Mrs. L. ends up saying, "I hate
you . . ." [Staff]

Mrs. Small [the older disabled person] accuses her husband [primary
support] of upsetting her so much that she had a stroke. They had a
fight about a bill that morning. His loud voice also upsets her. He stays
out late—goes out, three to five evenings per week; sometimes he
doesn't come at all. He had a girlfriend who died last year. Mrs. Small
says he treats her like a child, tells her what to do. [Staff]

Strained relationships also developed among family members over the allocation of responsibilities and the failure of some members to appreciate the contributions of others. One woman said, "If I start to do anything for my mother
she wants more and more." Some other case studies illustrate further problems:

Basic themes in contacts between the primary support daughter and
FSP caseworker include the daughter's resentment of her care-giving
role, her resentment and anger toward her brother who refuses to become involved, her anger at her mother for accepting her son's lack of
involvement. [Staff]

It has created problems between me and my brother. He's married to a
woman who will not cooperate. She and I will not speak to each other.
He feels like I'm forcing him to do things he doesn't want to do. . . .
He feels that I shouldn't ask her to do anything, that I happen to be
married to a nice, easy-going guy and he's not married like that and
what can he do? He's not going to force her to do anything.

Mrs. Fisch's suggestion that Mr. Fisch place his mother was one reason
for their legal separation. [Staff]

Relationships were also strained when the older person and the supporting
family member could not agree on how much or what kind of service was
needed.

Wife: He shouldn't lift heavy grocery bags.
Husband: I only carry light loads and I enjoy it.

We had to argue her into getting a cleaning woman. She thought housecleaning was good for her and it kept her limber.

In these situations, the older person typically wanted fewer hours of homemaker
service, and the other family member wanted more. Sometimes disagreements
between supporting family members and the elderly were of great significance.

The doctor said to put my mother in a nursing home. We looked around
for one and made it on the waiting list. Well, she got sick over it. She

said she wouldn't go. When the home finally called, my mother answered the phone and said she was no longer interested.

After she broke her hip, we twisted her arm and she agreed to go to a nursing home, but she never went. I've got the nursing home papers in, and as soon as I have her certified, we are just going over there and get her out of her apartment.

Motivation, Burden, and Impact

What motivates families to maintain such levels of support for the functionally impaired elderly in the community? Families in our study were guided by a sense of indebtedness, the fear of nursing-home placement, or both. These families did not usually receive practical or financial help from their disabled relatives. Family members rarely cited reciprocal service and aid exchanges with the disabled person as a strong motivational force. In the absence of contemporary exchanges, families are usually motivated by their sense of indebtedness. They may feel as if it is something they have to do, though it does not make them happy, or that they must do it because of the family connection. One woman said, "I'm obligated to do these things since I'm her daughter, but I really love her." Another case was described in this way:

> She said that her mother had always taken care of her, made her lovely clothes, and worked very hard. She was determined that she would take care of her mother to the end of her days. It was evident, however, that this was a great strain on her physically. [Staff]

Fear of nursing-home placement is a frequently cited motivation, usually expressed with emotional intensity, as in one family who had placed the older person in a home but later decided in favor of home care: "I'd go out there [the nursing home] and see them all lined up against the wall. I couldn't stand the abuse. That's why I took him home."

Families may maintain their disabled elderly at considerable financial sacrifice. It is very difficult for a supporting family member to obtain financial assistance to cover the costs associated with serious functional disability. This applies most directly to elderly couples or siblings who live on fixed incomes and must finance unusual medical and/or personal care expenses out of limited resources. It also applies to adult children who have their own household and family finances to manage:

> If there is something I need, I can get it, except money. I tried welfare, but all they deliver is help. I don't understand why they don't give me the money they are going to give someone else. I've got nothing left. I can't buy myself anything, not even panty hose or earrings.

The most difficult thing for me to do is pay the bills. Finding the money
is difficult to cope with. After my husband's heart attack he developed
a terrible cough. We had to go to a specialist once a week and it cost
$10 just to get there and back in a taxi. We owed $800 to the doctor. I
took out a loan to pay the doctor bill last year. Now I owe the bank
$800, and I've already overspent this year.

Long hours and considerable frustration appear to be inescapable burdens
for families who are motivated to maintain their disabled elderly in the community. Job interruptions, restricted freedom, less time for recreation and
enjoyment, and pressure to carry out a certain number of supportive activities
in a limited amount of time dominate the lives of family care givers.

It's the time element. Everyone has to have a little time to himself in a
twenty-four hour-period. She can't be left alone for a minute.

I have no time for myself. I can't plan ahead. It's hard to get together
with my friends. . . . I just wish I had more freedom.

I used to like to go downtown and go to a restaurant or to a show, maybe two shows, but I can't do that now.

Mr. Jones began to explain that he kept a night job while his wife
worked in the day so that there would be some member of the family
around in case his mother needed them. He talked of doing the shopping, paying bills and checking in on her. In addition, since she could
not get to the bathroom, it was necessary for him to empty the commode. [Staff]

Families experienced various hardships as a result of their reponsibilities for
their aged relatives. Some family members attributed specific physical ailments
that they had developed to their care-giving responsibilities.

It affects me quite a bit. It gave me high blood pressure. Can you
imagine your mother being as active a woman as she is and seeing her
slowly deteriorate—wouldn't it affect you?

He [primary support] has occasional flare-ups of high blood pressure.
"She's [the older person] overbearing, although she doesn't mean to
be. She just is. He [her husband] has been having flare-ups in his
pressure. She has the attitude that everything is due her." [Staff]

A middle-aged sister quit her job; a granddaughter dropped out of school; an
adult son reportedly left his wife because she insisted on nursing-home placement for his mother. But family members most frequently complained about
regimentation and restricted freedom. This burden is made even more profound
when the family perceives there is no relief in sight in the future. In long-term

care of the disabled elderly, the burden of care appears to be forever. The families already had long histories of providing service at the time of contact with the program. Said one, "There's no end. . . . I'm extremely tired most of the time. . . . It's the routine, all the time. . . . It's the routine."

Rather than expecting relief from their roles, primary supporting relatives feared increasing dependence:

> I returned to school in January. . . . At the time I made the decision she was coming along fine, but I didn't change my mind when she went into the hospital. I went on to school. If anything worse would happen I'd just drop out.

> My brother is very concerned and upset about it. He has not related any fear, but he's very anxious because each setback is making her more dependent.

Each person in the family network seemed to have a threshold of support beyond which he or she found it difficult to increase supportive activities. This threshold of support varied greatly for individual family members. For instance, an aged sister lived a short distance from the older person and did her cooking and shopping; however, she did not want to increase that level of support by moving in with her sister.

> She said having her sister move in with her would be signing her own "death warrant." She said her sister's present needs and demands were overwhelming and that if she were to move in with her, these demands on her time would double. . . . There are other relatives, but they work, have families of their own, and do not live nearby. [Staff]

> Quite frankly, it was very debilitating, as though it were too much. I'm working full time, have a house to run, and seeing her every day took its toll on both of us. I knew I had to stop going every day.

> Mrs. Stone [the primary support] explained how last year she had been caring for her husband and sister at the same time, had developed twisted intestines, and did not take the time to get any help for herself until she suddenly ended up in the hospital. That's when her brother and his wife had no choice but to come and stay with Mrs. Cunningham, which they did. The day Mrs. Stone returned home, immediately Barney and his wife left, not even remaining for coffee that Mrs. Stone had offered. Mrs. Stone is very angry at him and she described this instance as one example of his overall attitude. She said she prefers him not to become involved. . . . She'd rather leave things the way they are. [Staff]

Even at the low and moderate levels of support, similar thresholds appeared.

> Mr. and Mrs. Glenn came once a week to visit. He keeps looking at his watch and they leave after exactly one hour.

Mrs. Reese reported that her son . . . was also worried. She thought we [FSP] would ask him to visit more than once every other week. [Staff]

The rationales for these thresholds sometimes seem insubstantial, however:

Her sister-in-law who lives in Brooklyn will come and spend the week-end with her mother. . . . The sister-in-law is not very fond of their dog and therefore will not stay for more than a weekend. [Staff]

That family members provided care did not mean that support was fixed. It could be withdrawn at any time, for a variety of reasons:

Their niece, who used to provide part-time companionship service five days weekly, obtained an evening job. Now she works at night and can't help in the day. [Staff]

The daughter, previously living in California, has been staying with her parents for four months until she finds a place of her own. "We don't want to get into a routine with her because it's temporary. We can go out sometimes during the week, but there's no point getting used to that."

Well, it depends on mother's condition and rate of deterioration, if it continues or accelerates. It might be that we'll be physically unable to cope, and we'll have to look for another arrangement. We are coping at the moment.

In some ways she has worn us down. We get tired of it. You can't feel pleasant and do it. . . . We've been talking about a nursing home, but we just can't decide. We don't know, but we don't want to be responsible for her going down, but eventually we know it's going to happen.

There may be a tendency in the professional literature on "natural supports" to over-estimate the number of friends and filial participants providing concrete care on a daily basis. In FSP cases when such support was required, the major portion of care usually fell upon one or, at the most, two individuals rather than upon a familial network. In the case of aged couples, the primary support was lo-cated in the same household and was probably retired. In the case of an indepen-dent household, a daughter usually took on the majority of tasks, or the male children of the older disabled person shared the supportive role with their wives. Other available relatives were outsiders in the family care network. There may have been token participation, but they provided little assistance with concrete tasks within the home. They played the role of a friendly visitor.

Summary

Most of the categorical and limiting conditions traditional to the public sector have been superimposed on home-care programs. For this reason, descriptive accounts of family support provide a picture of service style and content quite different from the predominant service configuration in home-care programs. Family members were able to concentrate personal care services in the early morning and late evening when the need for such care was greatest. They provided a diversified mix of services that included heavy and light housecleaning, personal care and housekeeping, shopping and exercise. Families also gave continuous service, such as twenty-four-hour-a-day supervision and companionship. They provided small units of service (an hour or two at a time), and they responded promptly to emergencies. They helped with residential relocation services, transportation, money management, and other finances. They did odd jobs such as snow shoveling or fixing a leaking faucet. Diversity and flexibility were the predominant characteristics of family care.

Services delivered by formal organizations and financed through public expenditures tend to be neither diverse nor flexible. Coverage restrictions are a convenient and frequent cost-control device. Services such as money management are subject to cumbersome legal regulations due to the risk of abuse. The regulations make the conservator and guardianship service costly and difficult to obtain. Inconvenience and higher costs are disincentives for any services provided on short notice, for a few hours only, or before or after the conventional 9 a.m. to 5 p.m. work shift. Professional tradition appears to explain the exclusion of residential relocation services. Public benefits for home care do not include cash transfers. The conversion of service benefits into equivalent-value cash transfers obscures a public-sector distinction between income maintenance and welfare services. When conversion of service to cash is allowed, a loss or reduction in accountability over public expenditures results. While some rationales for narrowly defined services appear more reasonable than others, they constitute serious obstacles to accomplishing greater flexibility and diversity.

How much broader should public-sector coverage be? Is it desirable for public funding and formal organizations to approximate the diversity and flexibility of the family support model? For cultural and legal reasons, the family will always operate with greater freedom than will the formal provider; however, organizational service characteristics might more closely resemble the style and content of family services. For example, present organizational distinctions between housecleaning and personal care functions can make delivery of both to the same client cumbersome. The family support pattern demonstrates that the specialization is artificial and functionally unnecessary. Family experience indicates that continuous supervision and incidental home maintenance are as crucial as they are difficult to obtain. To be effective, public programs will need to assume some responsibility for these problems. They will need to develop an evening, night, and early morning service capacity similar, perhaps, to the way hospitals organize shifts to provide continual coverage.

When home care is provided by both a family and an organization, it is reasonable to expect coordination of their functions. When families are incorporated into the definition of client, as in the FSP, potential conflicts of interest emerge in coordination. Not all family members agree among themselves about the best service strategy. In some instances, family members and the older person disagree. In the absence of consensus within the family, whose perspective should prevail in arranging outside services? It was not uncommon for service staff to be asked to arbitrate or take sides in resolving family service disputes. Family members occasionally requested a meeting with the worker in order to obtain the professional's cooperation in overcoming the disabled person's objections to family preferences for services. This placed the service staff in a precarious position. The family's cooperation with the service plan is crucial, but in obtaining cooperation, the staff may take actions objectionable to the older person. At a minimum, public policy should assert the right of disabled older people to refuse intervention and services they deem undesirable. Service agents of the public sector should be obligated to comply with the older adults' service (or nonservice) preferences even at the risk of neglecting what the family or staff may perceive as needs. Such a policy would also require incompetency procedures comparable to those now employed in probate courts.

4

The Domain of Service

In an attempt to encourage family persistence, FSP offered primarily a combination of home care, public entitlement advocacy, and professional supervision with counseling. Home care was funded either through New York City programs or the project's own budget. FSP had no authority over public programs but assisted families in acquiring benefits. FSP staff also monitored home-care quality. They directly supervised home-care workers employed by CSS and had some leverage over home care through purchase of service agreements with homemaker agencies in the city. At the time they entered the program, eighty-three families had or acquired homemakers. CSS financed service for fifty-eight of them and directly provided the homemaker for twenty-one of the fifty-eight. Homemakers' services were limited to a maximum of thirty hours per week. (See table 4-1.) Medicaid financed care for another twelve cases. In the course of the program, Medicaid and the New York City's Human Resource Administration (HRA) became an important source of care. The home attendant, homemaker, and housekeeper are the city's major programs. The home attendant program is intended for those with the most severe disabilities, requiring the most extensive care. In 1979, the home attendant program served 21,600 cases and provided an average of fifty-two hours of home care per week. Persons requiring less-extensive care were served through the housekeeper and homemaker services, which had 15,300 and 2,600 adult clients, respectively, in 1979. Other resources for home care include New York City's Department on Aging Title 3 funds and the department's own homemaker program.

Table 4-1
Home-Care Provider and Source of Funds ($N = 83$)

	Percent of Families
Source of funds	
FSP	69
Medicaid	14
Cost sharing (FSP and family)	11
Families only	6
Home-care provider	
CSS	25
Outside agency	63
Relative, neighbor, or friend	12

In 1978, expenditures for the three HRA programs totaled $152 million. Expenditures for hospital- and community-based home-health agencies in New York City that year came to $47 million. The magnitude of New York City home-service expenditures can be appreciated when compared to national data. In 1977, national public home-care expenditures totaled $1.13 billion. In the following year, public home-care expenditures in New York City alone totaled $178 million.

The FSP staff also counseled family members and the impaired elderly, provided advocacy on behalf of the impaired person with other public programs, and provided general case monitoring. The standard combination of advocacy and monitoring in the long-term care field is now identified as case management, although the term was not used by the staff at the time. The FSP had the opportunity to combine case management with the direct authority to purchase or supervise home care. Counseling overlapped both therapeutic and management functions. Therefore the program was able to scrutinize service arrangements closely.

Home Care

The homemakers were the crucial direct-service component of the FSP. Eighty-six percent of the families (eighty-three) received home services on the average of 11.6 hours per week (see table 4–2). Homemaker service was usually organized into half-day intervals with the typical family receiving three half-days of homemaker service per week. The more-impaired aged clients were likely to have more than four hours per day of homemaker service (see table 4–3).

Table 4–2
Home-Care Level of Benefits (N = 83)

Frequency of Benefits	Percent of Families
Days per week of service	
1	13
2	34
3	22
4–6	26
7	5
Hours per day	
4	62
More than 4	26
Less than 4	12
Hours per week	
Less than 8 hours	21
8 hours	25
12 hours	21
13–25 hours	18
Over 25 hours	15

Table 4–3
Homemaker Hours per Day, by Functional Impairment Score ($N = 82$)

	Four Hours or Less		More Than Four Hours	
FIL Scores	Number	Percent	Number	Percent
0–5	21	34	1	5
6–11	19	31	3	14
12–17	9	15	5	24
18 and over	12	20	12	57
Total	61	100	21	100

Home-care workers performed the usual functions of housekeeping, shopping, meal preparation, personal care, escort, and so on (table 4–4). The most frequent services were light housekeeping and marketing. Forty-five percent of the families received personal care. Because of the difficulties in purchasing a combination of housekeeping and personal care, it is likely that the frequency reported here reflects constraints in supply as much as assessed need. The interrelationships between receipt of personal and other home-care options are shown in table 4–5. In examining the overall distribution of home care, it is obvious that there is a relationship between level of impairment and hours of homemaker service, with greater impairment associated with more hours (table 4–6).

Introducing a homemaker into a household produced mixed results. In some instances, the intimate nature of the homemakers' work resulted in very close and personal relationships with the disabled person, and the actual tasks performed were well integrated with the support that family members provided.

Table 4–4
Distribution of Homemaker Functions

Type of Service	Percent of Families with Type of Service[a]
Light housekeeping	84
Marketing, shopping	72
Meal preparation	59
Personal care	45
Companionship	43
Escort	42
Assistance with feeding	20
Exercise	10
Administering medication	6
Money management	0

[a]Percentage total is greater than 100 because many families received more than one service.

Table 4–5
Interrelation of Personal Care and Assistance with Transfers, Escort and Companionship, and Light Housekeeping (N = 82)

	Personal Care Provided	Personal Care Not Provided	Total	
	Percent of Total	Percent of Total	Number	Percent
Assistance with walking or transfers				
Provided	31	17	40	49
Not provided	14	38	42	51
Total	45	55	82	100
Escort				
Provided	21	22	35	43
Not provided	24	33	47	57
Total	45	55	82	100
Companionship				
Provided	20	23	35	43
Not provided	25	32	47	57
Total	45	55	82	100
Light housekeeping				
Provided	39	45	69	84
Not provided	6	10	13	16
Total	45	55	82	100

She [the homemaker] keeps the place immaculate, does sewing, cooking. . . . She reads to her sometimes. It's a fond friendship. Laundry, ironing—they both work together. [The homemaker] will let her do a certain amount.

I have a nice home attendant. Just to show you . . . my mother says she likes Bertha, but that she combs her hair *too* much!

She looks forward to her coming. She hates to be alone. She can't always remember who the home attendant is, but she knows she's quite fond of her.

The homemaker goes to the library, cooks, shops for food. . . . She makes a meal at night, makes the bed, any little thing mother asks. On nice days, she takes Mr. F. outdoors and they sit in a neighborhood park.

Other family members obviously benefited from relationships of this type between the disabled person and the worker. In part, they felt more secure knowing a dependable attendant was present. They were also relieved of some obligations.

Table 4-6
Degree of Functional Impairment, by Hours per Week of Homemaker Service

	Less Than Eight Hours		Eight Hours		Twelve to Twenty Hours		Twenty or More Hours		Total	
	Number	*Percent*	*Number*	*Percent*	*Number*	*Percent*	*Number*	*Percent*	*Number*	*Percent*
Low disability (total FIL < 11)	11	25	18	41	11	25	4	9	44	100
High disability (total FIL > 11)	5	13	4	10	15	38	15	38	39	100

Note: $\chi^2 = 17.91$, $df = 3$, $p < 0.001$.

It's a relief when I know someone's going to be there every day 'cause I'm very worried when she's there by herself.

At least we know that someone is coming in on those days. Just the feeling of knowing someone is there that day. She can take a bath, and the homemaker will do the tub and tidy the place. Just someone being there and talking to her.

When the primary supporting family member was also disabled or frail, homemakers performed tasks that could not otherwise have been accomplished.

I can't do it myself, so naturally, it helps. It helps because I'm not able to do anything. I can't do it and my wife (who is legally blind) can't do it, so it's got to be helpful in that respect.

When the primary supporting family members worked full time, a home-maker service created new opportunities for free time by releasing them from some household chores. The result was, as one family member referred to it, "a new peace of mind." In some cases, the staff encouraged family members to make use of occasional respite for temporary relief from their own commitments to the disabled person.

Mrs. Cunningham explained how her husband had been very ill last year and she was left with the responsibility of caring for both her husband and her sister and now "feels trapped" and needs to get away for a weekend. No one else in the family will take over the caring and she doesn't know what to do. [Staff]

A primary support husband and his disabled wife were given a two-week vacation at a summer camp.

They called me immediately after their return. They told me that "every-thing was perfect, the food, the people, the entertainment, etc. We never expected it. We never had such a good time in our lives before." . . . They talked about camp ever since and were happy when I told them they could go back this year. The experience really gave them a lift which lasted, even with Mrs. Leanard for quite sometime. [Staff]

Seventy-five percent of the family members receiving respite opportunities were the adult children of the disabled person. Respite was offered to families in particularly trying circumstances. It was here that the FSP services were most flexible. Such expenditures were consistent with the service as incentive philosophy fundamental to the project and constituted an imaginative use of funds. This raises an intriguing public-policy question: if one purpose of a public program is to relieve temporarily the overburdened family member of responsibility, then should the purchase of recreation and entertainment with benefit dollars be permitted? If it is permitted, what restraints, if any, are to be established?

Family members also appreciated the attention that disabled elderly received from the homemakers because it often reduced the older person's demands for emotional support:

> The home attendant keeps her busy. We work and must take care of the house, shopping, washing. . . . When we're home, we can't entertain her. She loves attention but we can't give it to her the way the home attendant does.

Sometimes family members reported improved relationships with disabled elderly as a result of homemaking help:

> Mother isn't as demanding. She gets many of her needs filled by the homemaker and therefore gets the best of us. She has a greater sense of security and feeling of still being in charge of her life.

Attempting to establish and stabilize service within the home was not always a smooth process nor was it always productive. The turnover rate among homemakers per family is one measure of the problem. Of those with a homemaker at the end of one year of service, only 31 percent had the same homemaker and 25 percent had had four or more (table 4-7). There is no external standard for judging homemaker turnover rates, so it was not possible to determine whether the FSP rate was unusual or particularly good or bad in comparison to other programs. The rate, however, appears high considering the importance that families attribute to a reliable and personable homemaker.

Homemakers might be removed or leave of their own accord. Personal incompatibility with the disabled person, failure to appear regularly on schedule, and incompetence were reasons cited for dismissal.

> The first homemaker was not satisfactory as she would not show up on the appointed days and would not call. After three weeks of this, Mrs. Lindquist called me and I reported this to the homemaker agency. [Staff]

> She was not sensitive and attentive, and could not cook well. I then hired a person from another agency, but the worker left the same day

Table 4-7
Homemaker Turnover Rate (*N* = 80)

Number of Homemakers Serving Single Family at End of First Year	Percent
1	31
2	28
3	16
4	25

because Mrs. Goldstein felt she was too young, and she refused to clean. From 12/30 to 1/21 a homemaker from a third agency was assigned and complaints were fewer. [Staff]

Mrs. Shaw advised that the homemaker had become very undependable and that she is positive she stole $40 from her. [Staff]

Homemakers sometimes found the older persons' or the families' demands unrealistic. Sometimes the physical circumstances of employment were too unpleasant, or there were personality clashes. In other cases, homemakers quit when they retired or found a better job.

Mrs. Felician had five homemakers in two weeks. These women had found Mr. Felician too heavy and difficult to maneuver for bathing, etc. The agency had male workers available but Mrs. Felician did not feel this would work because of his paranoia about her and other men. . . . She contacted the homemaker agency and was told no other women would consider the position. [Staff]

Earlier, the homemaker and Mrs. Todd were having difficulties. Ms. A. describes them as a problem of communication and personality. The homemaker wanted to "take over" and Mrs. Todd resented this. [Staff]

Mrs. Fisch watched the homemaker at all times. When she went into the kitchen or bathroom where she couldn't see her, Mrs. F. would call out to her, "What are you doing?" She also asked her constantly if she had finished this or that chore yet. When she sent the homemaker to the store, she made her read the shopping list out loud first and scrutinized every item in the bag when the homemaker returned. Though she complained about a few things, she didn't send her back to the store because the homemaker had to do other chores, but I understood that she often does send the homemaker to exchange things.

The quality of the home-care component proved to be extremely important to client satisfaction. As one family member said,

As soon as you began to get accustomed to them, they left. I think there were three, possibly four. They all did their work quite well, but I felt it wasn't good like that to have someone coming into your home and building up a relationship and changing, saying, "Tomorrow someone else is coming." They shouldn't change so often; elderly people don't accept changes too quickly.

The rate of homemaker turnover varied with the type of provider (table 4-8). In comparison to the homemaker services purchased from other agencies, the turnover rate among CSS homemakers was relatively low. Thirty-five percent of the CSS homemakers were still with the same family at the end of the first year, whereas only 18 percent of the homemakers from other agencies were with the same family. CSS homemakers were long-term employees of the agency and participated in the same fringe-benefit programs as did all other agency personnel. Similar employment benefits were not generally available in homemaker agencies, so CSS was able to offer more-attractive employment to workers. To some extent, the turnover rate at CSS was attributable to the expansion of the homemaker staff. As new homemakers were added, some clients were reassigned to the new staff. For example, a bedfast client was reassigned to a male homemaker who would be able to do the heavy lifting that was required. When friends and relatives of the aged person were hired to perform homemaker functions, they had a lower turnover record than did either CSS or the other homemaker agencies. Fifty percent of the employed friends or neighbors were still on the job at the end of the first year.

The problems in securing long-term, reliable, and companionable homemakers appear to be seriously underestimated in long-term care policy and program planning. FSP directly administered a small percentage of the home care that its clients received. The staff had little to do with the selection of homemakers provided by other agencies or the city. More expansive and thorough demonstrations will need to create and test a work environment that makes homemaker jobs more attractive. If high-quality, dependable employees are to be retained over a long period of time in homemaker positions, jobs must be competitive. Issues in homemaker recruitment, selection, salaries, benefits, career opportunities, training, assignment, and supervision are central to a successful home-care program.

Entitlement Advocacy and Case Management

Thirty-two percent of the FSP families received assistance in obtaining and monitoring public entitlements. Assistance primarily dealt with Medicaid applications and home-care benefits available through the New York City HRA

Table 4–8
Homemaker Turnovers by Type of Agency ($N = 64$)

Number of Homemakers, First Year of Service	CSS		Purchased Outside		Friend or Relative	
	Number	Percent	Number	Percent	Number	Percent
1	7	35	7	18	4	50
2	5	25	12	32	1	12.5
3	3	15	6	1.6	2	25
4 or more	5	25	13	34	1	12.5
Total	20	100	38	100	8	100

programs. From income information obtained during the FSP application procedures, staff members were able to determine potential eligibility for public
benefits.

Decisions about whether to make an application were sometimes complicated, and some families were grateful for information about public benefits and
assistance in applying.

> I'm very grateful because I would never have known about the Medicaid
> services. It was the social worker that sent in the application to the
> City. So you see what your agency has done for me? I could never
> praise them too highly.

Other families were reluctant to apply for such services, for a variety of
reasons. They were skeptical about the quality of care; they were reluctant to
spend down (relinquish to the state) assets of income in excess of the maximum
stipulated in eligibility standards; they feared having too much care forced upon
them; they were philosophically opposed to accepting public assistance; or they
resented the intrusiveness of the public bureaucracy.

> Mrs. Stein has declined to apply as she wants to keep her saving intact
> for her burial. [Staff]

> The HRA worker had upset her by telling her she would have to accept
> a significant amount of homemaker service in order to get Medicaid.
> Mrs. Butts herself is not sure how much service she needs. . . . She does
> not want to slide and let others do everything for her. She does not feel
> she could tolerate it. [Staff]

> The possibility of making an application for SSI and a Medicaid home-
> maker was firmly rejected. Mrs. Smith (the older person's sister) said
> that the financial assistance she gave her sister was not a hardship for
> her, and accepting welfare was out of the question. [Staff]

> (Since Mrs. Smith would never declare in writing that she would no
> longer support her sister financially, there was nothing I could do in
> this respect at this time, especially as Mrs. Goldstein's rent is $298 per
> month, which is not acceptable to SSI or Medicaid. [Staff]

There are significant costs associated with pursuing and securing public
benefits. Bookkeeping, documentation, and in-person filing requirements for
application and recertification are very demanding. Spend-down eligibility
required perpetual recertification. Also families always risked unanticipated
decertification and payment problems, which would disrupt the flow of service
and exaggerate the application costs. Another problem was that HRA checks
for home attendants were sometimes held up or sent to the wrong address. The
client paid the home attendants with a two-party check from HRA made out to
the attendant. When the home attendant was replaced, the client often received

checks made out to the previous attendant. An HRA worker explained to the staff, "It takes six to eight weeks for a change in name to take place."

The project staff advised everyone who was eligible to apply for Medicaid or Medicaid spend-down. Of course, when families received publicly funded, substitutable home care, substantial reductions in the FSP budget resulted. This is not an unreasonable cost-containment strategy on the part of a private agency. The home-care budget for FSP had a fixed ceiling, so when the public sector assumed the home-care costs for a family, FSP resources were freed to enroll new families or provide more care to present cases. Another result, however, is a potential conflict of interest between families and staff. The project could reduce costs (or enroll new clients) by using Medicaid financing whenever possible, and families could reduce their costs by using FSP home-care workers and refusing Medicaid workers. Generally there were fewer service disruptions and better supervision with the FSP homemaker staff.

> I made it clear to Mrs. Inez that if she needs more time from FSP, we could not pay for this. She would have to go on Medicaid. [Staff]

> We're in the process of applying for Medicaid spend-down. The social worker advised us to start the ball rolling. I assume that if any additional FSP services would be available, she would have told us.

When the project required families to use publicly funded home care, it absorbed some of the families' costs. For example, FSP purchased homemaker service until application determinations were made.

> Mr. Fisch said he is in contact with Mr. Mann of HRA and has had spend-down explained to him. Financially, he said he is under a burden because he is really not able to pay for a private homemaker. I explained that our program's help would be available until an HRA homemaker could be installed. [Staff]

When clients were already receiving Medicaid assistance, advocacy services were provided to help the families comprehend HRA regulations and comply with them if possible. When an older person gave a check to a Medicaid home attendant for time she had not worked, the caseworker and family spent months trying to recover payment from HRA. In this same case the social worker also authorized a loan to the family until the matter was settled. The social worker also helped fill out and deliver forms for the annual Medicaid recertification.

> The social worker contacted me at the time of recertification. . . . She came over and helped with recertification forms and advice. I have always known there's someone I can call when I get in trouble.

> I contacted the surgical supplies who said a doctor would have to fill out form 40, in order for her to get a multiposition foot board. . . . She

needs a twenty-four-hour-a-day home attendant—which has been approved by Medicaid. This was not initiated due to the lack of another room in her apartment. . . . The family claims the Veterans Administration will not give enough money to cover a two-bedroom apartment, which would be necessary to institute live-in home attendant.

Other advocacy responsibilities involved securing food stamps and working with the Social Security Administration and hospitals:

Mrs. Jones had not received her social security check. On Feb. 3, she called the office on 125th Street, but the person who answered was rude to her and so she hung up and then called the office at 2 World Trade Center. She doesn't know if they will follow up. She accepted my offer to help her with this matter. I called the Social Security Administration on 125th Street, and they mailed her the card to fill out and sign about the missing check. Mrs. Jones received a replacement check within a few days. [Staff]

The social worker from the hospital has not called except once yesterday. It's through the FSP social worker that we get to know what's going on.

My mother did contact the social worker when she had difficulty with the landlord. It's a very good feeling to know that the agency can deal with officialdom in one way or another. The social worker was much more effective than we could have been.

As part of its management function, the staff assisted families with supervision of the homemaker. Problems with unrealistic family expectations or unreliable homemakers were widespread. To some extent, these problems appeared to be avoidable or remediable, and shared supervision between staff and families seemed to help. The staff members brought an independent point of view to structuring and evaluating the performance of the homemaker. They concluded that in some instances, ineffective homemakers had been retained too long by families unable to dismiss them, and in others, that families imposed unreasonable and conflicting expectations on the homemakers.

When no one party was obviously at fault, the task of finding and correcting errors required subtle judgments. For instance, in the Atwood case, a long series of homemaker placements was pursued, to no avail. Within two months, there were four different homemakers: the first was accused of sitting and doing no work, the second was accused of being too domineering, the third was accused of drinking and bringing in friends, and the fourth was dismissed for an unknown reason. After trying five more homemakers in the following two months, the daughter assumed these responsibilities herself until her mother could be placed in a nursing home. There appeared to be problems with all parties involved.

Some form of joint supervision among the family, the older person, and the agency appears promising and desirable, though it is not necessary in every case.

In many instances, family members easily supervised the homemaker. In the absence of problems, such supervision seems appealing since it is essentially cost free. But even in cases where great confidence could be placed in the family's ability to supervise, some program monitoring of compliance and quality would be required. Certainly levels of intensity in monitoring could be adjusted to complement family responsibility. There would be inevitable questions over standardizing such a procedure. Undoubtedly shared supervision occasionally would lead family and staff members to conflicting evaluations of homemaker performance. Under these conditions, the authority to hire, reprove, or dismiss homemakers might become controversial. Ultimate authority must clearly rest with either the project or the older person and family.

Who bears the burden of incompetence and the burden of detecting and remedying it? From a public-policy perspective, it is desirable to define the reasonable assignment and balance of management costs among the public sector, private agencies, and family members. The task of articulating policies and standards is complicated by the subtleties of quantifying nonpecuniary costs for family members. At a minimum, both family members and staff in FSP appreciated the advantages of cooperation in homemaker supervision. The more-serious responsibility for maintaining a backup service capacity that could be initiated in the face of unpredictable disruptions or chronic delays is more complicated. In FSP, the backup function remained the family's responsibility. Rarely was a staff member pressed into cooking a meal, shopping, or cashing a check when the homemaker did not appear as scheduled. The staff was adamant that emergency relief would not be incorporated into the program design. The policy question remains, however: should this be solely the family's responsibility? What emergency relief precautions, if any, should be taken for disabled elderly without families? The sheer size and sluggishness of public bureaucracies suggest that private-agency programs modeled after FSP would be a more-viable option for emergency relief. It is not obvious, however, that private agencies would leap at the opportunity to bear the burden of backing up the failure of public services to perform reliably; neither is it obvious that the public sector would be willing to finance such an operation or permit reimbursement of agency expenditures for emergency relief claims prior to formal eligibility determinations. If so, private agencies might perform the smaller but still meaningful role of consultant to the family.

Counseling

Counseling consisted of supportive casework, information, and advice about family care. Either the disabled elderly or their family members were the recipients of counseling in 42 percent of the cases. Counseling, which focused on coping with disability directly, or with a disabled family member, was provided to the older person in 15 percent of the cases.

Most of the time was spent talking about Mrs. Brice's upset and depression. [Staff]

Focus in counseling was in the following areas: life review, anger about her deteriorating health, and her increased feelings of self-worth as she becomes more adept in the use of her prothesis. [Staff]

My mother has been seeing a social worker for counseling for a marked depression experienced as a result of her sister's death from cancer and her recent diagnosis of cancer of the bladder. She wouldn't talk or eat or get out of bed or anything. She lost about twenty pounds. I knew it had to do with my aunt's dying.

The social worker was very helpful. If my mother needed someone to talk to, she could talk to her. It was that and financial assistance that was most important.

In 18 percent of the families, the primary supporting relatives received counseling. Some relatives discussed their roles in providing care and the support or lack of support offered by other family members. Some expressed guilt over not being able to do more or expressed resentment of their burdens and the demands that they felt were unreasonable.

They [the project personnel] know how to work with other people. I have a good sense to know how to work with older people, but sometimes you get puzzled. You don't know which way to turn and I always called FSP to get someone to give expert advice. They're a great help.

I've never had to relate to a handicapped person, and the social worker was used to this, so this was helpful.

When the social worker talks with me, all my burdens disappear. I feel so relieved. . . . She knows the stress I'm under. She suggested I go away. I will pay for a half-day practical nurse, and FSP will pay the other half.

I have an interview with the social worker once a month. If it hadn't been for her, I don't know what I would have done. We talk about my mother and different things, and what we talk about helped me a lot. She's a wonderful person.

The social worker has been in constant touch with us. Visits me and visits my mother and helped a great deal in helping me talk because I do feel guilty about what I am not doing. She says, "Look, you're doing all right." She understands me. . . . She was the one who told me, "Watch, your mother is playing games with you." It stopped when the social worker started talking to me. . . . I'm not so smart about old people's thinking.

Counseling was provided to both the older persons and the primary support in 9 percent of the families. It was usually offered to the older persons and/or the primary support in the family meeting. In the mutual agreement letter, the social worker usually wrote, "I would like to come and talk with you about any concerns or problems you may have," or "I will be available to you for counseling about any worries and concerns you may have with which I may be of help." Sometimes the workers were more aggressive in offering counseling services.

> Previously, I had suggested on the phone that she needed to develop a new attitude toward her back condition and that she and I could discuss this difficult adjustment over a period of time, in hopes that she would come to feel a little bit better. [Staff]

> I confronted the B's with the fact that there seemed to be some problem in how much care they were giving Mrs. Schechter and how this was affecting their own life-style. I gave permission for their having a life of their own and thought this was an area in which we could be helpful to them, namely, counseling. [Staff]

Some families resisted the offer of counseling, either rejecting it explicitly or just not using it. When questioned, one natural support daughter seemed offended, and answered very coldly, "I don't feel this counseling is necessary."

The workers attempted to describe the nature of their visits in terms that would be most palatable to the clients.

> Mrs. Nachman and I made a definite arrangement for me to *visit* every other week. I clarified with her that I was not visiting because she needed counseling but that old age is a difficult time and most older people seem to want to express their concern to someone. [Staff]

> I said I would be able to be in touch with Mr. Jordan and the family periodically should they have any concerns they feel they want to discuss. Both children said they thought their father would "enjoy my visits" but did not seem to express a great need for regular home visits as long as things were working out well with the homemaker. [Staff]

Many clients did not seem to know whether the social worker's visits were intended as counseling or not. Said one, "Counseling? No other than the social worker who does come over once a month or so and talk to my mother about an hour or so. When the social worker can pay us a visit she does. She has been up a few times." Letters of service commitments sent to the families typically stated, "the social worker is available on a regular or periodic basis to discuss the problems you are facing," or "The social worker is available to discuss other concerns you might have." Not all clients interpreted this as a specific service assignment by the staff.

When the social workers conducted this counseling without client awareness, their professional roles sometimes took on a casual and conversational quality.

> I felt that Mrs. Nachman would prefer me to visit as a friend, even though she called me her social worker. Last time she wanted me to drink some tea, and when I refused she felt very rejected. . . . I went over with Mrs. Nachman that she had used my visits to talk over certain events in her life, but I wondered if she had wanted more than a good listener. She said no, she had a need to talk, a compulsive need, and now it was out of her system. [Staff]

> Mr. Jordan has used my visits to talk about his illness but usually prefers to discuss other issues of interest to him—in short, casework here has taken on more of a monitoring role with less need for more intensive casework involvement. [Staff]

Yet the workers felt these visits, in spite of their limitations, had some value for the older person. The visits could be reflective of a more friendly, supportive relationship rather than a professional-to-client relationship. One social worker explained, "In spite of Mrs. Crane's tendency to utilize interviews in this way, my visits serve as a means for her to express her feelings of depression over her situation."

The clients expressed appreciation for the personal friendship within the context of the counseling relationship.

> "My mother likes to be with young people in their twenties and thirties. She enjoys visits from the social worker. She likes to have young people around and it's lucky for her she has a young social worker."

> Mr. Reese says he's benefited from the service for he need not be the brunt of his mother's depression. His mother has benefited for she has an obsession with her illness, and anyone she has outside the family to talk about it provides an outlet for her. She can air her problems. [Staff]

5

Changes in Patterns of Maintenance

Families, the principal source of home care for disabled elderly, may regard the introduction of agency-based home care as a substitute for their own contributions. Substitution has implications for both the number of services that disabled elderly receive and the cost of home-care programs. It is assumed that some division of labor between the family and the state is reasonable, but another question is whether a modest service contribution can relieve families of some responsibility without stimulating massive withdrawal.

This chapter examines changes over time in the relationships among disability level, family contribution, and agency services. In general, the analysis describes the interrelationships in the one-year cohort (eighty-four families) and two-year cohort (48 of the eighty-four families in service for two full years).

Changes in Functional Disability

The response of family members to the introduction of service must be considered within a context of the changing level of need for assistance. Changes in disability provide some basis for estimating change in need for help. Fifty-one percent of the elderly in FSP had an increase in their Functioning for Independent Living score during the first year, and 54 percent had an increase in the second year. In both years, the increases in disability tended to be in the area of physical rather than mental functioning.

By the end of the first program year, the mean total FIL score increased from 11.6 to 12.5 (table 5-1). For those who remained in the program for two years, the FIL score increased from 11.0 to 15.9 (table 5-2). Increases were statistically significant. Thirty percent of disabled persons in the one-year cohort experienced substantial increases (four or more points on the FIL scale) in impairment, and 44 percent in the two-year cohort had similar increases. The following examples describe the families' experiences when disability increased.

> Mrs. Sherwood is an eighty-six-year-old widow who lives with her only daughter.
>
> FIL scale at program initiation = 3.
> FIL scale one year later = 10.
>
> Research interview after one year: Mrs. Sherwood's problem of a ringing in one ear began about six months ago. Her headaches have become

Table 5–1
Differences in Mean FIL Scores over One Program Year ($N = 83$)

	Scores at T_1[a]	Scores at T_2[b]	t Value
Total FIL	11.6***	13.5	-3.17**
Confusion index	4.1	4.0	0.06
Physical functioning index	8.7	9.6	-1.96*

Note: Higher score means increased disability.
[a]T_1 = program initiation.
[b]T_2 = one year of FSP services.
*One-tailed probability < 0.025.
**One-tailed probability < 0.001.
***Mean scores for confusion index and physical functioning index do not add up to total FIL because of missing data in confusion index for five cases.

Table 5–2
Differences in Mean FIL Scores over Two Program Years ($N = 48$)

	Scores at T_1	Scores at T_3[a]	t Value
Total FIL	11.0[b]	15.9	-4.07*
Confusion index	4.0	4.4	-0.36
Physical functioning index	8.8	11.5	-3.30*

Note: Higher score means increased disability.
[a]T_3 = after two years.
[b]These means differ from table 5–1 scores because forty-eight of the one-year cohort cases continued into and completed two years of service.
*One-tailed probability < 0.001.

more severe. Her forgetfulness has increased. According to her daughter, Mrs. Sherwood can have breakfast and five minutes later forgets she ate. She used to be able to clean floors, sew, and prepare her own breakfast. Now her daughter says she can only do dishes but then won't know where to put them afterward.

Mrs. Weber is an eighty-seven-year-old widow who lives in an apartment with her only daughter.

FIL score at program initiation = 9.
FIL score one year later = 19.

Research interview after one year: I notice that in every respect it's going down, down. She forgets. The other day when I called her, I was so happy she remembered your name. She used to be able to say "call this one" even if it were ten calls. Now I tell my friends, don't leave any messages. And she's weakening. She wants to go to sleep. As soon as she's had breakfast and everything, she wants to go to bed.

Mr. Wilson is eighty years old and lives with his seventy-eight-year-old wife.

FIL score at program initiation = 11.
FIL score one year later = 17.

Research interview after one year: He's bent down and falls very often. He was hospitalized for a month to six weeks in January of this year for a fall he had taken in the house. He had a fractured pelvis in January. He fell in the house. At first I didn't think it was anything, but I called the doctor that Friday night and he said, "I don't know what it is, but I don't think it is a fractured hip." By Monday he was in agony. I took a cab and took him into the hospital. He stayed a month and then he came home with a walker.

Only 14 percent of the older persons experienced substantially improved functioning in one year. Over two years, only 11 percent reported similar gains.

Mrs. Smith is sixty-eight years old and lives with her seventy-one-year-old husband. She suffered a stroke before she entered the program.

FIL score at program initiation = 7.
FIL score one year later = 3.

Research interview after one year: Mrs. Smith no longer needs help entering and leaving her bed, chair, or toilet. She still requires help in the bath or shower and needs help in getting in and out of a car. [Smit]

Mrs. Clarke is an eighty-nine-year-old widow who lives with a daughter and granddaughter. She is confused.

FIL score at program initiation = 24.
FIL score one year later = 18.

Research interview after one year: She is now able to perform most transfers with the exception of a bath or shower. . . . She can handle her dishes and move a chair, but she can't hold items weighing five pounds or more. If she gets to the commode in time, she will have no accidents. . . . Mrs. S. reports that her mother's health is improved.

For 56 percent of the elderly, there were only slight changes (from one to three points) in the FIL score after one year. Forty-four percent of the elderly had no more than small changes in the FIL score over a two-year period of time.

Mrs. Jenson will soon be ninety years old. She is widowed and lives alone.

FIL score at program initiation = 3.
FIL score one year later = 4.

Research interview after one year: "Changes? None with the exception
that she did have a fall. She was going to sit on the bed and stepped on
a needle and went to sit on the bed and missed it." . . . Her daughter
did not feel that the fall was serious enough to warrant a hospital visit.

Changes in Agency-Based Services

Services provided by FSP tended to change over a period of two years. During
their first year, eighty of the eighty-four families received some homemaker
service. Fifty-three percent of these families had increased homemaker hours in
the first year, and 30 percent of the two-year cohort had increased hours. Forty-
one percent of the families in the first-year cohort had no change, and 64 percent in the second-year cohort had no change. The remaining 6 percent in both
cohorts had reduced homemaker service. Over the two-year period, there was
some leveling off in frequency of service expansions and in requests for increased
service. Although 46 percent of the family supports reported requesting additional service in the first year, only 27 percent of the families said they requested
additional service in the second year.

Corresponding to this overall change, there was also increased use of Medicaid-financed home services. Fourteen percent of the elderly received Medicaid-
financed home-care service after they entered the program. Thirty-eight percent
had such service after one year in the program, and 45 percent of families still in
the program after two years had it. When families became eligible for Medicaid
home services, they tended to get more hours of service than FSP had provided
directly. Ten of the thirteen families (77 percent) receiving Medicaid homemaker
service during the first year received an increased number of hours. In fact, for
five of the ten families, there was a forty-hour per week increase when FSP's ten
hours were replaced with Medicaid's fifty hours of service. Eight of nineteen
families already on Medicaid at the time of enrollment in FSP had similar substantial increases in the number of Medicaid-financed homemaker hours. Medicaid's capacity to finance care was greater than FSP's, and there is no reason to
assume the two programs followed the same criteria in determining benefit levels.
For example, one case with a very low disability score received five full days per
week of home care. Unpredictable variation in public benefit levels can usually
be attributed to the applicant's social characteristics, demeanor, and level of
disability, as well as the discretion of the assessment specialists in the public
agencies.

The availability of external funding becomes so important as a causal factor
in change in service level that any direct relationship between change in disability
and service level and between service requests and service level is potentially
distorted. Nonetheless, it appears that requests did have an effect on service
expansion. Seventy-one percent of those requesting additional service in the
first year received it (table 5-3). There is a statistically significant relationship

Table 5-3
Family Requests for More Service during First Year, by Change in Level of
Home Care ($N = 80$)

Change in Home-Care Level	Did Not Request Additional Hours		Requested More Hours	
	Number	Percent	Number	Percent
No change or fewer hours	27	64	11	29
More hours	15	36	27	71
Total	42	100	38	100

Note: $\chi^2 = 8.62, p < 0.01$.

between requests and service change in both cohorts, although the relationship is
weaker for cases during their second year. In the second year, 58 percent of
those who requested more service received it (table 5-4).

Among the forty families with increased disability in the first year, 55 percent received increased hours of home care (table 5-5). During the second year,
essentially the same pattern continued, but with a slightly weaker relationship
between increasing hours and increasing disability (table 5-6). This response is
less direct than it appears, however, because 53 percent of the entire sample
received increased hours of home care during the first year. The same pattern is
evident when a distinction is made between those with slight increases in disability and those with substantial increases. Once again half of the latter group
received increased service. From each of these perspectives, the relationship
between increasing disability and increasing service is weak.

There were other changes too. As part of the initial service package, 26
percent of the families received homemaker service for the purpose of respite.
Thirty-three percent at the end of one year and 45 percent at the end of two

Table 5-4
Family Requests for More Service during Second Year, by Change in Level of
Home Care ($N = 47$)

Change in Home-Care Level	Did Not Request Additional Hours		Requested More Hours	
	Number	Percent	Number	Percent
No change or fewer hours	28	85	5	42
More hours	7	15	7	58
Total	35	100	12	100

Note: $\chi^2 = 4.58, p < 0.05$

Table 5–5

Change in Level of Disability during First Year, by Change in Home-Care Hours (N = 79)

Change in Home-Care Level	Same or Decreased Disability		Increased Disability	
	Number	Percent	Number	Percent
Less or no change	19	49	18	45
More hours	20	51	22	55
Total	39	100	40	110

Table 5–6

Change in Level of Disability during Second Year, by Change in Home-Care Hours (N = 47)

Change in Home-Care Level	Same or Decreased Disability		Increased Disability	
	Number	Percent	Number	Percent
Less or no change	16	76	17	65
More hours	5	24	9	35
Total	21	100	26	100

years received homemaker hours for respite. Over time, the number of contacts between family members and FSP social workers declined. On the average, social workers contacted the older person or family members once a month throughout the course of the program. Thirty-eight percent of the families at the end of one year of service and 16 percent in the second year received case-work counseling. FSP staff provided entitlement advocacy to 40 percent of the families during their first year of service and to 20 percent of the families in their second year of service. Special escort service, heavy housecleaning service, and financial help with recreation were provided by the end of the first year in 36 percent of the cases and in 48 percent of the cases during their second pro-gram year.

Changes in Supportive Capacity of Family Participants

In the analysis of substitution effects, change in family capacity is an important intervening variable. In FSP, only 6 percent of the families had a decline in the number of participating members in their first year in service. Seven percent reported an increased number of participants. During the second year, only 4 percent of the families had fewer supporting members, and 8 percent had more. These small changes suggest relative stability. Also the primary support member was replaced in only two cases over the life of the program.

The functional levels of family members were not tested, but there is qualitative evidence that in a small number of cases, there was dramatic and conspicuous change in the ability of a primary supporting member to continue at the same level.

> I had an accident. I fell in the elevator shaft and broke one leg, sprained my back. . . . I can only drag around the house. I walk with a stick.

> The doctor says I must have done something, wrenched my back or something. Every move is an agony like a sudden stab in the back. I try to avoid it by moving very slowly. I'm hopeful that it'll go away sooner or later.

In the absence of a backup capacity within the family, such changes resulted in less support.

More often responsibility was transferred to other family members, and in two cases at least, greater responsibility was shifted back to the member originally designated as disabled. For example, a niece took care of her disabled aunt when her uncle was hospitalized, and a daughter provided an escort service when her elderly aunt could not continue.

> I had a mastectomy last September, and I've been very depressed. . . . Since I had my operation I haven't done much. He [the disabled husband] took over the cooking, but I'm doing it now. I do my cleaning now. I have to renew his medicine. . . . I remind him of things.

> Mr. Green had to have a pacemaker because of a serious heart condition. He is improving, but his ability to do many little things is impaired. Mrs. Green now attempts to do more of her own personal care because of her husband's health. She still is able to fix her hair with one hand, as well as sew. [Staff]

The subtlety of these shifts makes the measurement of capacity quite complex and vulnerable to unreliability. In FSP, qualitative data imply that overall family capacity is relatively stable even if difficult to measure precisely.

Changes in Level of Family Support

Over 60 percent of families both in the one-year and two-year cohorts reported no change in the level of support they gave. Central to the question of substitution is the frequency with which families provide less support. Twenty-three percent provided less during the first year and 15 percent provided less during their second year (table 5–7). Even if all of these cases could be considered straightforward withdrawal, the substitution effect is not large. Furthermore, both qualitative and quantitative evidence indicate that factors other than substitution are related to a reduction in the level of family support. Some reduction is part of a larger pattern of fluctuations in support. For example, of the thirteen families who did less in the first, ten (77 percent) reported no change in the second year. Of the twenty-seven who reported no change in the first year, only four (14 percent) provided less support in the second year. Three (6 percent) of the total forty-eight families reported doing less in both years. While twenty-three percent of the families reported doing less in the first year, 23 percent also reported doing more in the second year (table 5–8).

In some cases the reported reduction was a deliberate part of the service plan. Family members sometimes were encouraged to do less. In fact, 25 percent of the cases received increased homemaker hours for the purpose of respite. In a sample of fifty-five cases in the first year, families reported the frequency of their activities in the Family Activity Scale (FAS). The mean frequency for the two years was essentially unchanged ($X_{\text{time 1}}$ = 56.2, $X_{\text{time 2}}$ = 58.6). The pattern overall appears to be one of basic stability with low-level fluctuations.

Table 5–7
Change in Level of Family Support, First Year and Second Year

Level	By End of First Year		By End of Second Year	
	Number	Percent	Number	Percent
Less support	19	23	7	15
No change	52	63	30	62
More support	12	14	11	23
Total	83	100	48	100

Table 5–8
Fluctuations in Family Support, First Year by Second Year

Changes in First Year	Changes in Second Year			
	Less Support	No Change	More Support	Total
Less support	3	10	0	13
No change	4	15	8	27
More support	0	5	3	8
Total	7	30	11	48

To explore the questions of substitution further, it is informative to examine the bivariate relationships between reduction in family support and changes in disability levels and homemaker hours. In both the one-year and two-year cohorts, there is no observable relationship between change in level of disability and reduced family support (tables 5-9 and 5-10). Overall the relationship between change in family support and change in disability was not statistically significant in either the first year (table 5-9) or second year (table 5-10), but it was in the expected direction. There was, however, a statistically significant relationship in the first year between reduction in family support and increase in homemaker hours (table 5-11). The pattern is identical in the two-year cohort (table 5-12). Thirty-six percent of those with more hours in the first year did less, whereas 10 percent of those with no change or fewer home-care hours did less. This pattern also appears in the second year.

Among the families who reported a decreased level of family support, many nevertheless remained extensively involved in the care of their disabled relatives.

> What I do? Decreased as far as cleaning is concerned. Cooking, I still help her as much as before. Before, I used to have to clean two apartments. So, it's much less. Cleaning is really the bulk.

> Relief? Definitely, I'd have to do my mother's housework and my own. It helps relieve me of extra work. I still cook for my mother and that ain't too bad, but the cleaning is hard to do, especially with little children.

> Sometimes I go to bed at 1:30 a.m. after a day of some cleaning and taking care of him. I feed him, massage his feet, give him the bedpan, and sometimes I have to hold the urinal if he can't. I have to cut his toenails and cut his hair and cook for him. I'm terriby tired and I needed a little help myself. It's the number of years I have taken care of him myself. Until FSP came along, I had to do everything.

Family members who did less nevertheless were likely to affirm their strong commitments to continued support.

Table 5-9
Change in Level of Family Support, by Change in Disability, First Year ($N = 83$)

Level of Family Support	Same or Decreased Disability		Increased Disability	
	Number	Percent	Number	Percent
More support	3	7	9	21
No change	27	66	25	60
Less support	11	27	8	19
Total	41	100	42	100

Note: $\chi^2 = 0.02$, $p > 0.05$.

Table 5–10
Change in Level of Family Support, by Change in Disability, Second Year
(N = 48)

Level of Family Support	Same or Decreased Disability		Increased Disability	
	Number	Percent	Number	Percent
More support or no change	19	86	22	85
Less support	3	14	4	15
Total	22	100	26	100

Note: $\chi^2 = 0.23, p > 0.05$.

Table 5–11
Change in Level of Family Support, by Change in Level of Home Care, First
Year (N = 80)

Level of Family Support	More Home-Care Hours		No Change or Fewer Home-Care Hours	
	Number	Percent	Number	Percent
More support	5	12	6	16
No change	22	52	28	74
Less support	15	36	4	10
Total	42	100	38	100

Note: $\chi^2 = 7.00, p < 0.05$.

Table 5–12
Change in Level of Family Support, by Change in Level of Home Care, Second
Year (N = 47)

Level of Family Support	More Home-Care Hours		No Change or Fewer Home-Care Hours	
	Number	Percent	Number	Percent
More or no change	10	71	31	94
Less support	4	29	2	6
Total	14	100	33	100

I do a little less, but my time belongs to her because we are both
widows and she is all I have left.

I love my mother and would never, never part from her. Nothing would make me stop taking care of her. My mother is my life now.

Family members would adopt new supportive activities that were less intensive, but complemented the homemakers' activities.

My telephone calls? It's down to once a week. Previously, I would call my father two to three times daily and spend the entire day off with him. Now the homemaker comes one day a week for five hours to dust and mop. She also talks to my father.

With the service I do less, except for fixing breakfast. And no more cleaning and that sort of thing. . . . I used to call two or three times a day. Now the homemaker calls me if anything goes wrong.

Some families did more rather than less during their enrollment in the program. Fourteen percent of the primary family supports reported an increase in their support during the first year of participation, and 23 percent reported increased support during the second year. In the first year of program participation, 45 percent of the families who did more also received increased homemaker service, and 55 percent did not. In the second year, however, 76 percent of the families who did more received the same or fewer hours of service (tables 5-11 and 5-12).

In some of these cases, the eligibility of the disabled elderly for certain publicly financed services had expired. For instance, when Mrs. Grant was no longer eligible for visiting nurse service, family members became more involved with her personal care and housekeeping activities: "We have been there much more often. . . . We have to empty the commode, make the beds, clean, sponge-bathe her, do the marketing."

Many of the families who did more were responding to the elderly's declining functional status. Nine of twelve families who did more during the first year of participation (75 percent) had relatives with increased disabilities. In the second year, 54 percent had relatives with increased disability.

He's gotten weaker. His speech has gotten worse. He has gotten more incontinent. He needs more attention. You had to feed him. Recently, I fed him completely—like his vegetables and soup. I had to feed him.

Lately she has trouble managing even simple finances, and I have to visit more and more. Now, I usually go once during the week, not just on weekends, to deposit a check or something.

My wife supervises her bathing now and rubs her down with bath lotion. My mother has to be dressed. We cut her food so she can eat. She's like a two-year-old now. Before, we fed her, told her to do her hair, but now we have to do it for her or direct the operation. We try not to do everything for her, to keep her more independent.

I have to wash her now. There was a time when she'd ask to wash herself, but I gave up on it. It was time-consuming watching her. I get up at 6 a.m. to do it. She used to wash herself.

Summary

The majority of families did not reduce their level of support in response to service introduction or incremental expansion of service subsequent to entering the program. Of the 23 percent of families who did less, most had received additional agency-based service. The staff encouraged families at high levels of support to do less by offering homemakers as respite. In only three of the forty-eight families followed for two years did the level of support decrease in both years. The substitution effect appears to be of a very low order and in many instances a socially desirable consequence of the introduction of service. Certainly families did not think of their short-range reduction as being inconsistent with their unaltered commitments to continued care. The account of terminations in chapter 2 also supports this conclusion. It appears reasonable to think that short-range substitution does favor long-range persistence.

As conditions varied for individual families, aggregate support levels in the study population were as likely to increase as to decrease. Most of the families who did more had an older member with an increasing disability; however, the majority of families with an increasing disability did not change their level of support. When disability did increase, families were more responsive with additional service than were FSP and the public agencies. With the inevitable plodding and rigidity of a large-scale service bureaucracy, families are an important response buffer to abrupt and serious changes in disability, as well as small-scale fluctuations.

6

Provider Discretion and Family Preference

Within legislated budget limitations, the public sector assumes a responsibility for providing services that satisfy the preferences of eligible recipients. The failure of nursing homes to satisfy consumer preferences is one of the strongest arguments in favor of new home-care alternatives.

Although all agree that home-care options should be attractive to consumers, there is no consensus on who should have the authority to choose or assign them. How important is it for impaired persons, their families, or their representatives to have an opportunity to express their preferences? Do consumers and providers disagree over the benefit packages? When they disagree, what are the consequences of their differences of opinion? What is the best balance of consumer preference and provider discretion?

Previous chapters described the performance of the demonstration, the role of the family, and the effect of service incentives. The focus now turns to the actual process of family and staff negotiations. If families were given their choice among services financed by the program, what would they choose?

One of the central objectives of FSP was to expose the service preferences of the family. Too often user acceptance of available service is accepted as the best measure of need. In other words, service supply determines demand rather than demand directing supply. Although quantity and content are not entirely separable, the focus here is on the preference for service content within predetermined constraints on level of benefit.

The Professional Model

The FSP strategy is a variation of the professional model, which emphasizes provider authority and discretion. The professional with training and expertise is qualified to diagnose need and prescribe service intervention. Individualized assessment requires discretion over possible responses. Rehabilitation or cure follows upon initiation of intervention. The model assumes that the consumer readily consents to the intervention and is satisfied with the rehabilitative results in the absence of error, incompetence, or abuse. The professional is accountable principally to colleagues. Only they are qualified to judge professional work. Services are produced on a fee-for-service basis. Professional discretion is the key selection criterion.

As they have emerged in the public sector, long-term-care demonstration programs, in general, adhere to the professional model. Eligibility and service decisions are typically the prerogative of case managers, identified as professionals and diagnostic experts; they may be nurses or social workers by training. Receipt and content of services are determined by the professional's assessment of need, which involves the simultaneous and nonstandardized consideration of all relevant variables. The variables themselves are not fully specified. Assessment determines need and therefore benefit. The case managers also facilitate delivery and monitor the users and the producers. The major service restraint on individual cases stems from a need to restrain total expenditures. Limits are set on the number of homemaker hours per week that can be authorized. Unless the user is so disgruntled with provider-designated services as to refuse them, user preference is considered synonymous with provider discretion. User satisfaction is the responsibility of the case managers, who rely on their counseling and management skills.

The use of the professional model as a mechanism for distributing public benefits has been subject to criticism in the past. In Medicaid, discretion is criticized for its contribution to escalating costs. As a professionalized mechanism of social control, unregulated authority to distribute or withhold desirable goods and services results in coercion.[1] For example, Ferleger describes professionals' use of discretion over patients' elementary freedoms (to smile, to talk, to mingle with other patients) in a mental hospital as a means of controlling behavior.[2] Failure to achieve equitable distribution of benefits in public welfare programs is also attributed to both functionary and professional discretion.[3] Persons in similar conditions receive unequal benefits. Discretion creates another equitability problem when personnel recruit applicants who are likely to do well in service programs and reject the more troublesome.[4]

In spite of these problems, the replacement of all aspects of individualized assessment and the elimination of flexibility in regulation appear to be an untenable proposition. If public-program regulations attempt to cover every possible human condition of life circumstance, the immense volume of directives would be difficult to implement. And the possibility would always remain that response to some special circumstance was not clearly prescribed by the regulations. Lipsky cogently argues that when people are required to make decisions about other people, discretion cannot be eliminated.[5] Street-level bureaucrats, to use Lipsky's phrase, have discretionary authority in large-scale service bureaucracies because the very nature of service provision calls for "human judgment which cannot be programmed and for which machines cannot substitute." The challenge remains, then, to employ discretion as a means to assure sensitive service response that prevents coercion and inequitability.

The written program protocol for FSP directed staff to intervene "as little as possible in the actual decision-making while providing the necessary information for families to make intelligent, well-informed decisions." The program brochure and other public relations material, however, did not identify the family's decisive role in defining services that the program design called for. The service-selection-by-negotiation strategy represents an untraditional attempt to relinquish some professional authority to the user while maintaining the expertise and discretionary element of the professional model. The mechanism for advising and negotiating was the family meeting conducted by the professional at the residence of either the impaired elderly member or another family member. Ideally meetings would be attended by all the involved family members. Family members were told that FSP would finance a "wide variety of services." Written confirmation of service decisions was prepared by the staff and mailed to families.

Exercising Discretion

In some cases, the service-selection process appeared to be very straightforward. Families knew what they wanted, made explicit requests, and the FSP staff made an immediate and direct response.

> Well, earlier my mother asked for an increase in the amount of time the homemaker came. The social worker arranged an additional number of hours. I can't remember what the service was exactly, but I know she got everything she asked for. Then my mother went to the hospital. I called and asked for someone to come in and stay with my father all day and all night. He couldn't be left alone. The social worker arranged for that, too. And when my mother came home from the hospital, the time was extended to cover this too. My mother also asked for someone to come in once a month and do heavy housecleaning. I know she got that, too.

> Mrs. M. asked what I thought could help in the situation. I told her we didn't need anybody for heavy housecleaning. My wife and I could do that. What was more important was that mother be bathed twice a week and have someone to take care of her personal needs. The woman who comes in and takes care of my mother is the best thing that could have happened to us in this situation. She has the skills to do it properly.

> I don't know anything about the services. Nothing other than they have homemakers. That's all I wanted to know about, and I didn't ask about anything else. If they told me, I don't remember. I was just concerned about getting someone to come in and help me out.

In these illustrations, not only is the situation obvious and the family member explicit, but the requests were made for traditional services that the staff knew how to contract for or produce. Thus the requests themselves did not challenge staff ingenuity or conventions or impose unusual administrative burdens. Services were competently and promptly arranged by the staff. Considering the major problems in the public sector with service-response time lag, this is a noteworthy accomplishment. In cases that involve unforeseen family disruption such as hospital admission or sudden illness, prompt and dependable in-home service response can be crucial to regaining stability.

In many instances, however, preference and discretion were not so compatible. It appears that the personnel tended to offer services that were already at their disposal or professionally meaningful to them. Both homemaker service and counseling were repeatedly suggested to families. The service suggestion carried with it the implicit authority of the professionals' expertise.

> She suggested a homemaker to fix lunch but I really don't like a person messing around in the kitchen.

> She asked me immediately if we wanted a homemaker, and I told her we already had one.

> The service we are getting is fine. I told Mrs. M. we don't need anything else, even though she suggested someone to clean. I told her, I know what you're offering, but I only want what we need.

It could be argued the homemakers were recommended under the prerogative of professional discretion; recommendations were made only when the family failed to recognize the need observed by experts. But the examples of rejected offers suggest another interpretation. Staff members viewed multiple-function homemakers as an all-purpose and readily available solution. To some extent, this may be a plausible, prompt solution since many situations would conceivably benefit from the service. Such practices, however, underestimate the preference for services typically excluded from homemaker care, such as personal care or heavy-duty housecleaning, or combinations of such services that are difficult to arrange. For example, workers filled requests for supervision with the assignment of a homemaker unless the time required deviated from the standard nine-to-five workday cycle. Families who asked for early morning, late evening, weekend, or nighttime supervision were on their own: "Mrs. Radin said they hoped to have someone come in at night who would stay in the spare room. I [staff] said perhaps they could ask around the neighborhood or their minister."

If an already-employed homemaker could be induced to work an extra evening or weekend, FSP would pay. The staff, however, did not take responsibility for recruiting homemakers for unusual hours, particularly for live-ins. The staff had serious reservations about these situations because of the difficulty in locating such people and the responsibility for the uncertain consequences of hiring an unknown person.

Although the negotiations were more complicated, counseling apparently fell into the same pattern. The program did receive overt requests for counseling from families. Counseling was also engaged or at least recommended when the staff member observed abrasive family relationships and adjustment-to-loss problems or experienced resistance on the part of the elderly person (or spouse) to agreements made regarding their care with other family members.

> Due to the tension in the home I believe that regular [counseling] visits are important . . . and should be done weekly. [Staff]

> I wanted to talk to her about what she will do after her mother dies. [Staff]

It could be argued plausibly that counseling, unlike homemaker service, is a subtle service, and the need is best detected by expert judgment. The staff, for example, could anticipate benefits from it that the family could not. And indeed some families reported gratitude for counseling services they had received but not requested:

> Mrs. Harper responded quickly to the idea that I would be able to see her on a regular basis to talk with her about her concerns, saying, "That's good!" She has a great many concerns, and it appears that she could utilize a helping relationship to discuss these things with an outsider, not one of her children. [Staff]

Such comments suggest that assigned counseling can yield otherwise unrealized consumer satisfaction, and case manager discretion is justified. To the traditional practitioners, there is little new in such an assertion.

A closer examination of the content of the counseling encounter and the consequences of assignment shows that some families considered and appreciated the counseling as "friendly visiting" and not as a service:

> My mother likes to be with young people in their twenties and thirties. She enjoys visits from the social worker. [Staff]

> I said I would be able to be in touch with Mr. Hunter and the family periodically should they have any concerns they feel they want to discuss. Both children said they thought their father would "enjoy my visits" but did not seem to express a great need for regular home visits as long as things were working out well with the homemaker. [Staff]

An attempt to define or clarify the actual nature of the service is further complicated when the worker denies to the user that the purpose of the encounter is counseling but defines it as such within the program. One caseworker said, "Mrs. Lewis and I made a definite arrangement for me to visit every other week. I clarified with her that I was not visiting because she needed counseling." And sometimes the staff equated counseling with monitoring:

> Mr. Jordan has used my visits to talk about his illness, but usually
> prefers to discuss other issues of interest to him. In short, casework
> here has taken on more of a monitoring role with less need for more
> intensive casework involvement. [Staff]

The end result is confusion over the nature of the service and its purpose.
If labeling counseling as friendly visiting makes a useful service more palatable to
a severely distressed family or impaired person, then some obscurity could be
considered desirable. In these illustrations, however, counseling does not closely
conform to the image of a technical, sophisticated product provided only by
qualified experts. The argument in favor of professional discretion for therapeutic services is weakened by the staff's loose definition of the service. For
administrative purposes, counseling services must be distinguishable from friendly
visiting and administrative monitoring.

Families were not aware that they had selected counseling or friendly visiting as one service from among the variety offered.

> Staff: There is no counseling mentioned at all in the report. It's
>   a significant service.
> Researcher: Is counseling mentioned in the case record? Or is it men-
>   tioned in the mutual agreement letter?
> Staff: I'm not sure.
> Researcher: This is the difficulty. Does Mr. Goldfarb know that he is
>   receiving counseling?
> Staff: I would assume Mr. Goldfarb knows he is receiving
>   counseling.
> Researcher: According to Mr. Goldfarb counseling was *not* mentioned
>   as a service.

The written confirmation of counseling sent to the family stated, "We will meet
with you to discuss issues that may arise . . . concerning the service plan. . . . We
will explore issues and stress that may arise." This written but ambiguous confirmation of counseling disguises both intent and mere presence.

It is informative to observe how the negotiations can be managed to pre-
serve the ambiguity. On one occasion a researcher accompanied a service staff
member to a family meeting. The staff member discussed service options for
forty-five minutes and made provisional decisions on a homemaker and an escort
for medical care. As the worker was preparing to leave, she stopped to ask,
"Would you like me to come back and talk with you every other week or so?"
The case record showed that counseling, escort, and homemaker would be provided, but the offer was phrased so that the family would not consider counseling a negotiated service item. The family did not perceive that a choice in services
was at issue.

Casework monitoring should satisfy administrative needs for program
efficiency and accountability. The extent of monitoring is determined by

administrative protocol, not by therapeutic need. If counseling occurs within a monitoring format, it is a bonus for the client. Monitoring should be restricted by definition of function and by administrative regulation of its duration and frequency. The optimal level of monitoring remains an open question.

Requiring families to accept some services must also be viewed in the context of other negotiated service decisions. If counseling or homemaker service is offered when other services are denied, then a substitution has taken place. For example, a family member in one case clearly stated her needs. "I can't get her into a bathtub. She needs a bench so I can bathe her . . . she needs exercise." Since these items were never part of the negotiated services, and this client did not specifically request the counseling subsequently provided, it is unlikely that an informed choice had been made in favor of it over other alternatives.

Counseling focused on financial planning was provided to a client who had incurred substantial debts for the purchase of care for her seriously disabled husband. This client explicitly identified financial debt as her major problem. If she had had the choice, would she have selected instead of counseling a cash transfer (of monetary value equal to the cost of counseling) for the purposes of debt reduction? When apparently reasonable requests were refused, some families withdrew even when alternatives were offered. Mrs. Page was without heat and hot water. She requested assistance with relocation and was offered a home-maker instead. The daughter, who said, "You bring someone [a homemaker] in, then you got trouble," withdrew from the program rather than accept a service she did not want. In another example, the family withdrew its application when the service response was inconsistent with the request for relocation:

> I have no privacy. I really don't have my own room. I sleep on the couch in the living room. I resent this. I also find my mother very talky, and if I just want to look at a newspaper or if I just want to close my eyes for a minute, she'll talk. I would like to live by myself, but if I ever got an apartment, I'd want a door that I can close.

Sometimes other services were substituted for those requested. In one instance, a family asked for assistance with relocation so that family members could live closer together, but the staff thought a more plausible solution would be to pay the costs of commuting. Locating adequate housing in New York City is very difficult. The staff felt that any effort at relocation was unlikely to be successful, and therefore it was not attempted. Was consumer preference relatively well satisfied or relatively distorted by such switches?[6]

Answers to this question might lie in observing the family's attitude toward service offers. A service staff, however, no doubt would object to equating family disenchantment with distortion. Families might be disappointed by their own errors in service selection or generally unhappy with their state of affairs. Also, families with unacknowledged requests might offer no complaint. Many FSP families who remained in service expressed extreme appreciation for what they got. In their desperate circumstances, they were grateful for any relief. Even families who received no service or received offers apparently inferior to their stated requests showed satisfaction: "Even though the homemaker wasn't started, the program has helped me to think clearly. It is somewhere to get advice. If things get worse I could call again."

In the following case, a request for a physical therapist was rejected: "A physical therapist from VNS was exercising him. We have equipment from the hospital. He had gotten to the point where he could almost walk. Then the service ran out and he returned to being immobilized." FSP offered a homemaker and the family accepted this solution without complaint. Such clients do not report dissatisfaction, and therefore the measure of distortion would be underestimated. Apparent user attitude is an imperfect measure at best. Estimating macrolevel impact is another approach. If such programs as FSP were implemented on a national level and enrolled large numbers of persons, the volume of business would magnify these differences into highly divergent national programs.

It is also necessary to consider situations in which services are denied and applicants rejected. Mrs. Cost was considered a candidate for nursing-home placement. She was quite frail, eccentric and inhospitable towards homemakers and staff. Her apartment was infested with cockroaches, mice, and rats, and homemakers were reluctant to even enter it. Mrs. Cost, however, refused to go to a nursing home. The case was discussed in a service staff meeting, and no one recommended hiring an exterminator as a partial solution. The staff concluded, "Her problem is she needs nursing-home placement." The client became ineligible because the staff's patience was exhausted and because her problems were not answered by traditional services. The ultimate problem was redefined to be failure to agree with professional judgment.

A need for providing such items as wheelchairs, hospital beds, handrails, bedside commodes, and shower benches occasionally were discussed by the families and staff, but rarely was equipment purchased from FSP funds. Total expenditures for equipment and home maintenance amounted to 1 percent of the total FSP budget. Neither were any permanent home improvements financed by FSP. Sophisticated prosthetic devices, such as a hydraulic bodylift, useful for bathing and transferring, were not discussed at staff meetings or purchased for families. The professional staff was not accustomed to providing such items and tended to think of them as beyond the services offered. The staff was more likely to acknowledge equipment needs when Medicaid was a possible source of payment. For example, the staff helped one family apply for Medicaid so they could get ambulette service and in another instance assisted with a Medicaid application for the purchase of a wheelchair and a hospital bed. But in spite of the apparent need for these items, the staff did not offer to purchase them when Medicaid would not pay. It is not obvious from the data whether families were simply unfamiliar with prosthetics, did not want them, or assumed they were indeed beyond the tacit definition of the services offered.

Enumeration of service-domain components is not characteristic of the professional model in social services. Professionals prefer to describe their services as "comprehensive" or "coordinated" or "available in a wide variety." When such descriptions are applied to long-term care and entitlements, it is difficult to know what actually can be obtained with the designated benefit. The outcome of the service-selection process is linked to the definition of domain. When boundaries are unclear even to the provider, worker interpretation becomes important, and internal consistency and user equitability suffer.

Professional perspective made the staff sensitive to the presence of apparent pathologies in the family, a reasonable concern in a long-term care program. Granting assistance to truly incompetent families would lead to future, undesirable repercussions for the staff. Denying assistance to competent families, however, would have no further repercussions for the staff.

In FSP, the basis for assessing pathology was sometimes obscure. In the following illustration, the applicant was rejected after a family meeting, although the levels of disability and nature of the requests were comparable to those routinely accepted. It is not entirely clear that the conditions here actually warrant the denial of benefits.

> The daughter is extending herself beyond what seems advisable for her physical condition. She has a serious heart condition and has been hospitalized several times. . . . She is determined to care for her mother as long as possible. I did explain that the family would not be eligible for FSP.

Other cases were rejected when the staff thought the sons drank excessively, thought a sister was extremely manipulative, and when a middle-aged son lived alone in his mother's basement apartment and had no social life. These cases were otherwise similar to those routinely accepted.

Although the basis for rejection is obscure, the decisions seem to reflect an underlying attempt to minimize risk of involvement with unpredictable and unreliable family members. One of the first cases referred to the program illustrates the problems that emerge. Mr. Howard (the disabled client) had previously cared for his wife who was diagnosed as psychotic. When he came home from the hospital after a stroke, his wife would not permit anyone in the house to help, although her husband needed insulin injections. A staff member realized that Mr. Howard had started drinking excessively when she found him and his brother intoxicated at 10:00 A.M., empty liquor bottles, and a pail of vomit in the living room. The staff worked intensively with a niece, a son, and a social-work supervisor from the hospital to establish a homemaker service. The homemaker was thrown out three times, and finally discontinued by Mrs. Howard. Three weeks later Mrs. Howard was readmitted for psychiatric treatment after she appeared at the hospital with a black eye. The experience convinced the staff to terminate its efforts, however. In a subsequent case, an apparently mildly retarded son and sole family support took a calculated risk when he left for work and his mother remained alone in her apartment before the homemaker had arrived. The mother wandered out and was lost temporarily. The staff interpreted the son's action as "neglect and abuse" and rejected the family. A reasonable case might be made for the son's need to protect his employment, but the staff perceived pathology, and the threat of entangling circumstances discouraged providing service even on a trial basis. Program experience at the operational level demonstrated that the more-acceptable risk of eligibility error is in the direction of inaccurate rejections. Any home-care organization will have an incentive to evade the greater economic and emotional costs of unruly, unstable families and clients, a tendency that would be intensified when front-line staff carry the very high case loads typical of most public social-service bureaucracies. Economy in case-load management is essential in the public sector.

In the professional model, the burden is on the client or family to prove worthiness for service. In an entitlement model, the burden would be on the staff to prove unworthiness.

Exercising Preference

In general, family members played a less important role in selecting services than did the professional. As service negotiators, family members were not very aggressive. When they were questioned about what they had asked for, they responded variously:

> I didn't say anything about how often the homemaker came. I didn't want to abuse your generosity.

> I was told what I could get and was glad to get that.

> I didn't ask for anything. Ms. M. [staff] suggested it. I never asked for anything in my life. Ms. M. did ease my mind by saying I deserved it.

> The social workers came to see my mother and provided the service they thought was necessary.

Each of these illustrations suggests a different reason for the families' failures to assume more-assertive positions. These families were unaware of the unusual role expected of them and did not discern it in the case manager's introductory description of the project. The families assumed the passive patient role characteristic of the medical-model expectations.[7]

Families preferred to think of themselves as modest in requests rather than greedy. There were instances in which families offered, apparently at their own initiative to share costs, and refused offers of additional service. Families felt uncomfortably close to the specter of poverty.

> I know what you're offering but I only want what I need. Why spend money on us when someone else needs it more?

> I manage pretty good. I have a small pension that gets us by. Let the people who have less than us, who need it more, let them have it.

Families in this situation were not good investigators of home-care options. Novice home-care consumers apparently require extensive new information to make informed judgments.

The staff discussed neither costs of specific services nor the benefit levels allocated in other cases.[8] This is characteristic of the case manager and professional model. The staff observed that families frequently were successful at expressing their stress and describing their troubles but were often unable to articulate specific service preferences. When families in FSP did not articulate preferences, were they uninformed or informed but unable to decide and act? Retrospectively it can be concluded that a lack of detailed information on the content of the variety of services offered contributed to families' uncertainty:

> I had no idea before the meeting what I wanted. They told me what would happen if I wanted a certain homemaker agency . . . they'd send someone over. . . . I don't know what the wide variety is but I'd know if I saw them in action.

> Researcher: Did you understand that the program offers a wide variety of services?
> Family Member: Well, how wide?
> Researcher: Well, for instance, escort, companion, homemaker, household equipment.
> Family Member: Well, as far as I know, not that wide, not that wide!

> The program offers us whatever we might need. Not so much in terms of we do this and this, but the conviction that the program would help.

In a few instances, negotiations with families became greatly complicated when family members could not agree on the desirability or the amount of a specific service. The supporting members might disagree among themselves about what was necessary, or they might be united in disagreement with the impaired older person about the necessity of certain actions. As a consequence, initiation of service might be delayed. In one extreme case, the staff worked for eighteen months to overcome disagreements within the family regarding in-home care. The spouse and the disabled elderly person refused to accept the homemaker that the son and staff member had agreed upon.

These disputes resulted in staff alignment with one or the other factions in order to implement some service. The staff members felt that their expertise and knowledge permitted them to make proper alliances and implement services. There is some support for this position, particularly when the mental ability of the impaired person is in question. For example, an aged pair of siblings were reported to be living in filth, and refusing medical attention and the assistance of a cleaning woman. The neighbors were alarmed and wanted them removed. The daughter and granddaughter were frustrated and exhausted. The staff's alliance with the adult children appears pragmatic and reasonable. Such alliances may nevertheless lead to conflict with the older person's preferences. In one extreme case, the staff was aligned with the adult children in an attempt to secure the mother's nursing-home placement against her wishes. The frailty of the elderly woman, the decision of the children to seek a safer environment, and the need for improved housing were accepted as adequate cause for placement.

It is obvious that the professional is not free of conflicts of interests in these negotiations. There is an incentive for even community-oriented staff to find nursing-home placement acceptable when the problems are numerous and the solutions complicated. In FSP, the client was defined as the family, not the disabled individual, and in many community-care programs, families can be expected to act as agents for their disabled elderly members. These definitions may result in actions opposed by the disabled person when there is disagreement within the family. Although families can impose their decisions, long-term care programs should resist the dubious role of enforcer. Obviously the line between enforcement and recommendation for service will be vague, but two protections are worthy of consideration. The first is a statement of principle that would prohibit implementing any service opposed by the disabled, elderly family member. Second, a grievance procedure might be of some use as a protection for a disabled person.

Summary

The professionals' method of negotiating indicates a need for more-stringent user protections. It is important to retain some program discretion, especially for the severely disabled without agents. It is also important to protect users from distortion or abuse of preference. If some service assignment in the presence of unformed preference or even opposition is allowed, what protection ought to be established to prevent the unnecessary denial of services which appeal to the families?

A major commitment to information sharing is essential. A standardized display of service options with detailed descriptions of housekeeping, personal care, companion, heavy-duty housecleaning, home maintenance, counseling, escort, household modification, prosthetic equipment, transportation, financial aid, and assistance in securing specialty (medical and legal, for example) services would help to educate users promptly. Such a display might be expected to provide cost comparisons also. Because of the ambiguity in definition, it is particularly important that users understand the costs of counseling or case managers' friendly visiting when it is assigned as a benefit. Without standardized service displays, the novice and uninformed user cannot be a very successful consumer of long-term care services. Long-term care programs should be required to perform this education service as a prerequisite for receipt of public funds.

On the surface, this might appear to require a marginal adjustment in the professional model. It is, however, likely to find considerable resistance on both professional and political grounds. Control of information is, after all, a very successful device for social control.

More critical still, the data presented here imply that control over selection should be placed in the hands of the user, unless legal incompetence could be proven. The professional model permits the user to accept, reject, or perhaps modify diagnostically determined service decisions. A service-claim model would permit users to select services by shopping among providers and require programs to compete for the user-controlled benefits. If public agencies determined the cash value of public benefits assigned on the basis of disability (or other criteria), then preference would be restricted by level of benefit and the quality of the provider competition.

Benefit level and specified domain of allowable services or products remain important and not entirely separate issues. Others have argued for a wider agenda of in-home services than is currently available. That point is certainly supported by these data and does not require reiteration here. In fact, competition might encourage expression of professional discretion as a means of creating attractive services. In conclusion, if consumer preferences are to be highly valued in long-term care, then a service-claim model appears to be a more promising alternative.

Notes

1. Joel Handler, *The Coercive Social Worker: British Lessons for American Social Services* (Chicago: Markham, 1973).

2. David Ferleger, "Loosing the Chains: In-Hospital Civil Liberties of the Mental Patients," *Santa Clara Law Review* 13, no. 3 (1973): p. 447–500.

3. Jeffrey Manditch Prottas, *People-Processing* (Lexington, Mass.: Lexington Books, D.C. Heath and Company, 1979).

4. Peter Blau, The *Dynamics of Bureaucracy* (Chicago: University of Chicago Press, 1963).

5. Michael Lipsky, "The Assult on Human Services: Street Level Bureaucrats, Accountability and Fiscal Crisis," in *Accountability in Urban Society: Urban Affairs Annual Review,* (Beverley Hills, Calif.; Sage Publications, 1978).

6. There were occasions when the staff was prepared to offer more service variety than the family could take advantage of. For example, a double amputee did not want the door thresholds removed as suggested by the staff. The client lived in an apartment building and was not permitted to make "structural changes" without incurring the risk of eviction. Similar obstacles were encountered.

7. Howard Freeman, *Handbook of Medical Sociology* (Englewood Cliffs, N.J.: Prentice-Hall, 1979).

8. When the program financed home care, families were at least aware of the cost of that particular service. Families were responsible for the payment of CSS funds to the homemaker agency.

7 **Designs for Home-Care Entitlements**

As the United States moves toward a home-care entitlement for the chronically disabled, major policy questions remain unsolved. The FSP has provided an opportunity to probe these questions while emphasizing the relationships between the family and the state. Family assumption of home-care responsibility is so widespread that it must be considered a crucial factor in the development of long-term care policy. Yet decisions regarding the role of the family and the extent of its responsibility have not obtained the visibility and consideration they deserve. Furthermore, credible objectives, realistic standards, and plausible program designs have not been clearly conceptualized for the long-term care field in general. The process of planning and evaluating the FSP has made clear the limitations of conventional wisdom in this field. Therefore alternative formulations for design objectives and standards are recommended in the concluding two chapters.

Two-Tier Entitlement

The FSP is important as a demonstration because the two-tier entitlement policy may have appeal to federal policymakers; thus its feasibility must be evaluated carefully. One tier would provide complete personal maintenance care for impaired elderly without family support. For those with families, the second tier would provide very modest benefits to complement but not replace family contributions. The experience with FSP suggests that such a policy merits consideration. The project had no difficulty in locating families who were assuming substantial responsibility for an impaired older adult. In fact, a large number of inquiries were received after very little publicity about the program. The service applicants wanted to continue their role and welcomed help. Relatives expressed deep personal obligations to disabled elderly members and dreaded the specter of institutionalization. Families experienced severe restrictions and regimentation in life-style that made them desperate for assistance.

The impaired person and other family members generally did not object to open discussion of service needs at a family meeting that the staff organized. In fact, the family members appreciated the opportunity. There were instances, however, in which the family members could not agree among themselves about service needs. At times, supporting members disagreed with each other and objected to the disabled person's preferences. Unfortunately the FSP model does not prescribe any standard solution to such dilemmas other than withholding benefits until a consensus is reached. The problem resides in treating the family as the eligible unit. It can be argued, however, that any program design would encounter potential users who objected to procedures or refused assistance. In spite of this limitation, the programmatic concept clearly establishes relief of family as a legitimate social objective. Relief is granted, however, only if the family accepts the terms of the offer and the authority of the provider to determine benefits.

The staff was able to negotiate modest service levels with family members, sustain their participation, and avoid escalation of demands. Faced with uncertainty about available service options and about benefit limitations, family members acquiesced to provider instruction. The homemaker service unquestionably was useful to family members, as well as to the disabled person. Family members claimed that the introduction of service helped them sustain their efforts. Family members did understand and agree to continue their support as a condition of eligibility. It appears, therefore, that modest benefits reduce the disincentive effect that results from a more-generous program for those without family resources. It is important for benefits to be attractive enough to minimize the artificial dissolution of family ties so that older disabled persons can qualify for higher benefit levels available to those without family resources. It is hoped that family support benefits could be structured so that public costs would be manageable. If successful, the two-tier strategy should substantially reduce the aggregate cost of a home-care entitlement. A cost-suppression effect is the strongest argument in favor of the plan.

The prominence of the family variable, however, conceptually weakens the social basis for a home-care entitlement and leads to serious operational flaws. There is a public responsibility to provide an adequate and humane level of existence for those who must cope with serious and unalterable impairments. Therefore it is reasonable to defray the costs of their care among the members of society at large. Receipt of benefits is conditioned upon the presence of serious disabilities, in the same way that Medicare and Medicaid provide benefits for the eligible who suffer illness or injury. It is contradictory to argue for a disability-based entitlement and simultaneously to assert that families must assume principal responsibility. There is a risk that the contradiction would lead to a confusion of purpose in a national program.

In the United States, social insurance programs are much more palatable to the electorate than are public assistance and welfare. For this reason, it would be desirable if long-term care programs adhered as closely as possible to an insurance model of testing eligibility and setting benefits. An insurance model further emphasizes the direct disability-benefit relationship. Again, it would be difficult to argue that chronic disability insurance benefits would be paid only if family support was absent. For instance, Medicare, a comparable insurance plan, pays health-care costs of the elderly regardless of the presence or absence of family capacity.

In addition to the problems created by the conceptual confusion and contradictions inherent in the two-tier plan, there would be obstacles in implementation. Determining the presence or absence of family is not necessarily simple. Clearly a disabled older adult without known living relatives could be categorized as being without family, but other conditions are more difficult to define. The issue is not mere presence but the degree of capacity to provide, as well as the legal obligation to do so. Measures of family capacity might include the number of relatives, their geographic proximity, their competence, their frailty or disability, their willingness, the quality of their relationship with the impaired member, and the extent of their other occupational and familial responsibilities. This collection of variables cannot readily be summed up into a uniform measure of family capacity and obligation.

The inevitable inconsistencies can be demonstrated through examples from FSP cases. Since adult daughters frequently are the primary supporting relative, presumably eligibility decisions would be based in part on their role. Would an adult daughter living a thousand miles away be held as responsible as well as one living ten miles away? Would the required degree of responsibility be proportional to their geographic distance? What would be the proportions? Would the contribution required of a retired adult daughter be greater than of an employed adult daughter? Or should a lesser contribution be expected of the more-aged daughter? Would an adult daughter without child-care duties be required to accept greater responsibility than one without young children to care for? Would the numbers, health, and age of children be considered? Should the adult daughter who suffers ill health or disability be required to make a smaller contribution than one who is healthy? Should the health and abilities of the adult daughter's husband be considered?

A fully operationalized two-tier plan would need to assess each legally responsible relative, including the spouse, siblings, and other adult children, on these variables. Which of these relatives could in fact be held legally responsible when many states no longer even hold spouses responsible for the costs of nursing-home care?

Family members in FSP did not always agree among themselves about who should do what or how much. Sometimes they disagreed with the disabled person about service needs. Under such conditions, would the state choose among the responsible relatives and assign responsibilities?

It remains to be shown that family contributions could actually be enforced. Would family members sever their ties rather than tolerate imposed obligations they considered unreasonable? When the disabled person or a primary supporting family member moved away, would a shift to a more-generous benefit tier automatically follow? Would it be necessary to uncover the motivation for relocation? If family members were caught evading responsibilities, would they be penalized?

Attempts to measure and enforce family contributions would result in enormous inconsistencies and inequities. There would be no standardization in the distribution of benefits. Obviously the costs of collecting such a large volume of data on every applicant's family would be prohibitive. The unstructured case assessment and monitoring style employed in FSP was also expensive. And it would be vulnerable to wide benefit variations among programs and among staff within programs. If an ill-conceived and operationally flawed national entitlement design is the best that can be accomplished in an era of retrenching social services, then inaction and delay may be preferable to expansion.

A Maintenance-Model Approach

How should a home-care entitlement and a nationwide service industry be structured? Whether or not a two-tier design is adopted in the future, the question is pertinent. The FSP data do provide an empirical basis for anticipating operational obstacles in program designs similar to FSP and for recommending alternative solutions. Recruitment and eligibility, benefit levels, domain of covered services, management, cost control, and impact on beneficiaries are the basic components of public programs. The pieces must be assembled in a way that is functionally practical and internally coherent while meeting basic performance criteria for public sector programs. There is general consensus that public benefits should be equitably distributed, services should be of high quality, management should be efficient, and cost should be controllable. To some extent, these desirable characteristics must be balanced and compromised. For example, a program with intense service monitoring might produce high-quality care, but the administrative costs might be unacceptably high. A well-conceived program inevitably requires a sophisticated and delicately structured package.

In contrast to the professional model, which tends to be characteristic of community-based, long-term care demonstration, is a maintenance model. The model emphasizes user control of benefits and standardized determinations of eligibility and benefit level. It also relies more heavily on market incentives to control quality and production costs. The principles of diagnosis, etiology, treatment, and rehabilitation that characterize the professional model are only marginally relevant to the maintenance of the chronically disabled. The purpose of home care here is to maintain, not to rehabilitate. Rather than placing responsibility for determining need, level of benefit utilization, prescription, delivery, and case management in the hands of one professional, the functions are segregated and independently regulated in the maintenance model.

Recruitment and Eligibility

In federal public-entitlement programs such as food stamps, social security, Medicare, and Medicaid, a premium is placed on the equitable distribution of benefits. Theoretically uniform and consistent treatment of applications results in similar benefits for persons with similar characteristics and in similar circumstances. This principle is highly valued in the United States and rests on a constitutional commitment to equal treatment under the law. A serious commitment to equitable distribution of home-care benefits to the chronically impaired would be operationalized with recruitment plans that resulted in high application rates from potential beneficiaries and standardized and consistent assessments of eligibility. The maintenance model would require strict disability testing to determine eligibility. The presence, absence, or degree of functional impairment is measured, and eligibility and benefit-level decisions are based on predetermined standards. Standards would be set so that only the seriously and chronically impaired received service.

In some states, variations of disability tests are practiced in the form of nursing-home preadmission screening and assessment instruments for community-care programs. Many of these instruments are constructed however, so that functional impairment and diagnostic information are interwoven. Usually such instruments are identified as psychosocial assessment. They include not only impairment data but also information on the respondent's degree of cheerfulness, happiness, anxiety, agitation, gregariousness, and personal satisfaction with life. The assessment instrument becomes cluttered with variables, many of them inappropriate for disability testing. Lack of cheerfulness and gregariousness are personality traits, not indicators of functional impairment. It is doubtful that they should be among eligibility criteria for public programs.

Even when dimensions of impairment are valid, the indicators of performance are often ambiguous and subject to interviewer interpretation. For example, disability items are sometimes scaled as follows: "performs task adequately with no assistance," "performs adequately with assistance," "performs tasks adequately with occasional assistance," and so forth. The key words are *adequate, assistance,* and *occasional.* Consider a task like bathing. What is "adequate" bathing? Is the ability to take a thorough sponge bath independently at the sink adequate bathing? If it is considered inadequate, should it be equated with the inability to bathe at all? What does *assistance* mean? Is that a handrail or bathtub bar? Or is that an attendant who physically lifts the impaired person from the tub? If they are both forms of assistance, should they be equated? Finally, how often is occasional? Is it once a day or once a week? Does the meaning of the word occasional vary with the task? The use of words like *adequate, assistance,* and *occasional* leaves much opportunity for individual interpretation. Most, but not all, of that interpretation can be removed when concrete indicators replace personal judgment. Accomplishing this is not a serious methodological problem.

The means of administering the instrument is probably more important than the instrument itself. Consistent use of a measurement tool requires training. As the number of assessors increases, the error due to inconsistent interpretation inevitably increases. There is a risk of random inconsistencies in measurement. Therefore it is desirable to minimize the number of people administering the disability test. Perhaps more important than random error, however, is the risk of systematic distortion (or instrument corruption), which can result when the party administering the measurement has vested interests to protect. For instance, in nursing-home preadmission screening, the level of care available often dictates the score rather than the score determining the level of care. Any measurement tool would be seriously corrupted if it were administered by the service provider (or even the case manager) who had responsibility for a recipient's level of benefits and, therefore, the quality of care. The burden of securing care and the burden of withholding benefits cannot be given to the same person without resulting in measurement distortion and inconsistency.

With adjustments in present instruments and administration of assessments, disability measurement is an attractive basis for distributing benefits equitably. But the instrument should be very concrete and consist of a small and manageable number of dimensions. Furthermore, control over the administration of the test must remain organizationally independent of the service-delivery and case-management components. Eligibility specialists should be trained and directly employed by the government. This quite conventional idea is comparable to the separation of eligibility from service in welfare programs today.

Take-up Rates

The take-up rate is the percentage of apparently eligible persons in the population who apply for and receive entitled benefits. The application rate for a national home-care entitlement program could be somewhere between 25 and 95 percent of the eligibles. Variable take-up rates have profound cost implications. In a cost-conscious service era, a low take-up rate could appear attractive.

The take-up rate can be readily manipulated. The existence of long waiting lists, lengthy turnaround times on application decisions, extensive documentation requirements, retroactive denials, frequent recertifications, and a demeaning manner among eligibility workers will help to discourage applicants from enduring the eligibility process. If home-care programs can be administered without such informal, discretionary controls, they offer more promise as an institutional alternative. If services were in adequate supply, available promptly, and considered to be reliable and attractive by beneficiaries, hospital discharge staff, physicians in private practice, and others, home care would become a more credible alternative. For the sake of consistency and equitability in the distribution of benefits through public bureaucracies, home-care programs should be designed to encourage high take-up rates. For the sake of predicting and containing expenditures, eligibility should be regulated with strict and explicit criteria.

To attract potential applicants, entitlement benefits and eligibility criteria should be widely advertised in the mass media. Extensive and detailed information should be printed in brochures and widely distributed. Announcements should be carefully worded to include a list of covered services, a thorough description of disability-testing and benefit-reduction criteria, and instructions for making application.

Benefit Levels and Benefit Reductions

A maintenance model would also promise more-generous benefits to those with greater functional impairment. The principle of uniform treatment would be satisfied by setting predetermined capitation rates. The cash value of the benefit would be indexed to the level of disability. The degree of precision in scaling benefits would be determined by the best precision obtainable in a disability instrument that gave consistent results. The actual cash values would be determined by the political process. They would reflect the willingness of the electorate to pay for the maintenance of the disabled. Assigning a predetermined benefit on the basis of a disability score is a mundane chore for a functionary.

Predetermined benefit rates might be reduced by a fixed formula that takes into account the applicant's ability to pay (means test) and the capacity of the family to provide support. There are precedents for both inclusion and omission of means testing in public entitlements. Means tests are characteristic of the welfare programs but not insurance programs. It would be desirable for reasons of operational efficiency and public tolerance to structure home-care entitlement as an insurance rather than a welfare program.

Means tests typically measure assets and income. Experience with asset testing in nursing-home placement suggests it may be impractical. Pauperization is a politically explosive topic. It has been very difficult to detect or prevent asset transfers to family members. It is not clear that asset-related revenues have been worth the political and administrative trouble they cause. If income testing is introduced into a maintenance model, it should be done in a palatable way. In a disability program in which the cash value of the benefits is predetermined and fixed according to the level of disability, income above a maximum limit could result in a proportional benefit reduction rather than a loss of eligibility. Of course, this is comparable to the Social Security Administration's approach to income testing, which is required for all those eligible under the age of seventy-two. Although this model deviates from traditional Medicaid and welfare income tests, there are no inherent obstacles to the benefit-reduction model in a disability program with fixed capitation rates, and politically, it is more agreeable to users and to the aging constituency at large.

Family capacity has too many dimensions to permit testing for eligibility purposes. Furthermore, the norm of obligatory family contributions would also need to be defined. If there is some limit to the extent of family responsibility, how will it be measured and specified? Standardized assessments and norms appear unrealistic.

Covered Services

A maintenance model for a home-care entitlement would not promise all covered services to all beneficiaries. It would promise the opportunity to select from among covered services up to the cash-value limit on the benefit level. In FSP, families routinely either sought or provided a variety of services:

Homemaker services, including cooking, shopping, housecleaning and laundry.

Personal care services, including bathing, toileting, feeding, exercise, medication, assistance in walking, and companionship.

Prosthetic equipment and other supplies that contribute to the safety and independence of the impaired client.

Heavy-duty housecleaning and home maintenance that is beyond the capacity of the impaired client but periodically required.

Transportation, including only the use of conventionally equipped automobiles, taxis, and public transportation without restriction on destination.

Assistance with entitlements, including information and referral, and case monitoring.

Telephone security checks to ensure that a client's unanticipated illness, accident, or injury does not go unnoticed.

Assistance with personal bookkeeping and financial management.

Location of adequate shelter and the means necessary to accomplish relocation.

Case management.

This list constitutes an inclusive but defined domain of care for the maintenance of the chronically disabled. Medical and health specialty services provided under existing entitlements—physician care, skilled nursing, skilled therapies, and counseling—have not been included.

Benefit Payments and Case Accounts

In the maintenance model, services are claimed by users rather than assigned by experts. To ensure beneficiary control over selection, the cash value or benefits would be paid directly to the user. A benefit account would be opened with the public agency responsible for administering the entitlement, and beneficiaries would draw from their accounts for the purchase of the covered services they choose. The process for handling claims and reimbursement sometimes is defined as a voucher mechanism. The principle is similar to the administration of the food stamp program.

Once benefit levels were established by the government, professional expertise would not be required to diagnose the need to have floors scrubbed, windows washed, linen laundered, warm meals prepared, and so forth. In many instances, the need for such items reflects the beneficiaries' personal preferences. This argument is reinforced by the failure of experts to agree with one another in diagnosing the home-care needs of a particular case.[1] In FSP, there were notable discrepancies between user preferences and professional prescription. Assistance in shopping for home-care options among suppliers will be required by some or many disabled persons, but this function is not equivalent to diagnosis and prescription. Some users might desire comprehensive case management, and they would be able to purchase it, like any other covered service, from their benefit account.

Public confidence in the feasibility of home care rests in part on sound evidence that public money will be spent for the designated purposes and the products will be of reasonable quality. A case accountant role is necessary to provide public accountability for benefit expenditures. In the professional model, this function is one of many assumed by a case manager. For this reason, the term *case accountant* is preferred even though it may imply a narrower range of responsibilities than is intended. The case accountant would offer advice and information on where the desired services could be obtained and on the relative merits and costs of the various options. Case accountants would review claims on their clients' accounts. Claims could be made by local suppliers of covered service and equipment, by beneficiaries, and by individuals employed by beneficiaries to provide covered services. Case accountants would also monitor the quality of direct service. Management and counseling functions would be segregated. In the professional model, a home visit every other week may be good counseling, but this convention should not dictate monitoring procedures. Counseling is a treatment strategy. If it were a covered service, it would be purchased out of the benefit account.

The nature of the relationship between the case accountant and the user makes the line between advice and coercion potentially vague. The influence of case accountants will be great in cases when a severely disabled user has no family or agent other than the accountant. Therefore when service claims are substantially altered or benefits denied for any reason other than exclusion by regulation, some formalized denial-of-service procedure should be required. In addition, beneficiaries should have a mechanism by which they can initiate a review of denials. (Similar review procedures should exist for disability testing and other eligibility criteria.) Beneficiaries who find it difficult to work with one case accountant should have the opportunity to switch to another.

The maintenance model presumes that functionally impaired individuals are neither mentally incompetent nor pathologically irrational. The presumption will not hold true in every case. Beneficiaries may also be victimized by manipulative caretakers who do not act in their best interests. Reasonable case accountants and users may also simply disagree on interpretation of regulations. To some extent, disagreements can be expected as part of normal routine and are not indicative of program failure. In this model, the burden of proof for the right to deny service would rest with the agent of the state, presumably the case accountant.

Suppliers of Service and Equipment

In the maintenance model, users would be free to choose their own providers. It would be desirable for beneficiaries to have multiple sources of service from which to choose. Among the regular choices would be not-for-profit organizations, voluntary agencies, for-profit agencies, and self-recruited personnel, including relatives, neighbors, and friends. Whenever one sector of the service industry is being expanded, considerable debate follows over the designation of eligible providers. The competing providers seek to capture as much of the future service dollars as possible by claiming a superior service capacity; their income, jobs, profit, and prestige are at stake. The for-profit agencies claim efficiency and dependability. Their detractors claim that the profit motive leads to skimpy services and that the quality of care is subject to deterioration. The voluntary agencies claim high professional standards and objectivity in assessing need. Their competitors claim that administrative inefficiency and unnecessarily enriched service packages lead to unnecessarily high costs. Clients may be attracted by the reduced costs of employing an independent homemaker or attendant at minimum wage and avoiding all administrative costs. This might lead, however, to the employment of unqualified persons and might prove to be costly and cumbersome for a public agency to administer. Clients may prefer to "hire" family members and thus avoid opening their homes to strangers or being subjected to personal and intimate handling by unknown persons. Opponents to this practice argue that it is difficult to monitor cash flows and ensure that the designated services are actually provided. No clear advantage in quality of care belongs to any single source of service. For this reason, competition among all of them would be encouraged. Ideally producers would seek to attract beneficiaries with imaginative service packages and low fees.

It is clear from the FSP data that the nature of services obtainable from existing homemaker agencies is in need of great improvement. There were frequent problems with homemaker reliability and compatibility with the user. Home care could not be purchased for short, irregular periods or before 9:00 A.M. and after 5:00 P.M. A combination of housecleaning and personal care was difficult to find, and the fee was considerably higher than for housecleaning alone. There was no twenty-four-hour-a-day intervention capacity for emergencies. With such extensive limitations and flaws, homemaker agencies could not provide a credible alternative to institutional care, regardless of the level of funding that might be available. In either a professional or maintenance model, a more-sophisticated delivery organization is required. Undoubtedly it would be necessary for public agencies to define the required delivery capacity and to stimulate the formation of suitable provider organizations.[2]

In FSP, the employment of independent operators, including relatives and friends, yielded a generally high level of service. The flexibility and reliability of relatives, neighbors, and friends exceeded that obtainable from agencies. Presumably fees for independent operators with no overhead would be less than organizational reimbursement rates. Impaired elderly with families willing to supervise independent operators could absorb some administrative costs and obtain more direct service for each benefit dollar.

The suggestion that relatives, particularly a spouse, be allowed reimbursement at a reasonable rate for their services usually invites skepticism and sometimes alarm. Nonetheless, in a disability-based entitlement program, the exclusion of family members from reimbursement is difficult to defend. In a few FSP cases, a spouse or adult child was near retirement and might have preferred reimbursable home care as substitute employment. Judging from FSP data, concern over quality of care is more of an incentive than an obstacle for reimbursing family members.

Control of Case Management and Administrative Costs

Personnel salaries are the principal source of costs for home care. Personnel can be divided into two levels: direct production, and management and administration. Regarding direct production, the cost of employing a homemaker or a personal attendant is basically a matter of salary and benefits. Degrees of investment in fringe benefits, training, equipment, supplies, uniforms, and transportation will produce some variation in direct cost. The nature of the variables does make them subject to government standard setting, monitoring, and regulation. That is the easier part of cost control.

Unlike the direct costs, case management and other administrative costs will vary enormously and will be more difficult to regulate. It may be that 40 to 50 percent of a home-care agency's costs ultimately will be attributable to administrative expenses. For example, the Community Care Organization of Milwaukee County reported that indirect costs were 39 percent of total expenditures.[3] In FSP, indirect costs ranged between 50 and 60 percent of total expenditures. The final report for Triage, a Medicare-financed home-care demonstration, showed that over 50 percent of the expenditures were for indirect costs.[4] In one highly professionalized home-care demonstration project in Chicago, homemaker services are reimbursed at a rate of $12 per hour. Of this $12, only 40 percent ($4.75) is attributable to homemaker salary. The remaining 60 percent covers administrative costs, excluding bookkeeping, which is donated by a local hospital.

Each of these illustrations leads to the regrettable conclusion that an administrative cost rate of only 50 percent might be the best that can be achieved in these programs. But is it reasonable to spend forty to fifty cents out of every home-care dollar on administration of the project level, to say nothing about the expenses attributable to state or federal responsibilities for management?

In comparison to the professional model, there are potential administrative cost savings in the maintenance model. Since an eligibility specialist with a single, straightforward disability test could replace diagnostically oriented assessments by professionals, nearly the same purpose would be accomplished in less time and at a lower cost. The service-assignment function usually claimed by professionals would be assumed by beneficiaries who shopped among suppliers for home care. Those unable to shop for themselves would require assistance. A clear distinction between management and counseling would permit less-intrusive and less-expensive monitoring procedures. Presumably a reduction and a deprofessionalization of the middle-man role will reduce administrative costs.[5]

Many of the cost-control strategies adopted for nursing-home reimbursement may be applicable to home care. In the coming years, there may be rate ceilings, single invoicing, regulated profit factors, limitation on pass throughs, indexing, fee schedules, utilization limitations, rate reviews, recovery programs for third-party liability, and certificates of need for home care. These strategies have not always been as successful as expected in regulating nursing-home care. Taking greater advantage of market incentives in a disability program, however, could complement regulatory activities and perhaps reduce reliance on cost-control regulations altogether.

Summary

Attempts to measure, define norms, and enforce family contributions to maintenance of seriously impaired elderly would lead to inconsistent and inequitable distributions of public benefits. A two-tier design is unlikely to satisfy minimum performance criteria for public programs. Nonetheless families do respond to incentives and generally are willing to work with external actors on problems in providing care. Therefore a disability-based public-entitlement program that openly acknowledged and rewarded family support might be the best solution.

It might also be the most expensive solution. If there was explicit and full assumption of public responsibility in a disability-insurance model, it is unlikely that family members would continue to provide care without making the claims for reimbursement to which they were entitled. To control costs, disability-based eligibility criteria would need to be simple, explicit, and stringently enforced. Also disability entrance standards would need to be high. Only the seriously disabled would obtain access to benefits.

Middle-level management would be nonintrusive. With predetermined capitation rates and strict disability testing, benefit levels would be efficiently and economically determined. Counseling functions would not overlap with case monitoring. Case accountants would provide public accountability and assistance to users. Suppliers might be independent operators, existing homemaker agencies, or new organizations that can provide an expanded range of benefits. Beneficiaries would have authority to select from a clearly specified domain of covered services and choose the provider that they prefer. Measurement of quality would focus on actual service delivery rather than the licensing of providers.

Overall cost control would rely chiefly on regulation of demand for care. Authority to test disability and benefit levels would remain the prerogative of the state. Administrative costs would be minimized by reducing management authority and the extent of supervision and counseling of users. Entrepreneurial service suppliers would be encouraged to compete with existing agencies and independent operators. Suppliers would attempt to market their programs with low fees and attractive benefits. Cost limitations would not be achieved by mandating family participation in long-term care. Cost control would be realized by making benefits available only to those with serious disabilities. Further, programs would be designed to allocate resources directly to the impaired elderly and their families and minimize administrative intervention.

Notes

1. Alan Sager, "Learning the Home Care Needs of the Elderly: Patient, Family and Professional Views of an Alternative to Institutionalization," mimeographed (Waltham, Mass.: Levinson Policy Institute, Heller School, 1979).

2. Francis G. Caro and Robert Morris, "Personal Care for the Severely Disabled: Organizing and Financing Care," mimeographed (Waltham, Mass.: Levinson Gerontological Policy Institute, Heller School, 1971), and Francis G. Caro, "Expanding Options for the Personal Care of the Disabled Elderly," mimeographed (Waltham, Mass.: Levinson Gerontological Policy Institute, Heller School, 1971).

3. "Second Annual Report," mimeographed (Milwaukee, Wis.: Community Care Organization of Milwaukee County, 1979).

4. Triage, "Final Report, 1979," mimeographed (Plainville, Conn.: Triage Coordinate Delivery of Service to the Elderly, 1979). As a Medicare intermediary, Triage incurred administrative costs beyond those associated with just home care. Therefore an exact figure for administrative costs is difficult to compute.

5. States are moving toward vendorizing and a Title XX administrative model for home care. It is not clear whether the strategy solves the states' management problems or simply makes them less visible. If states relinquish to vendors their authority to test disability and determine eligibility, then conflicts of interest and slippage of the states' regulatory power would seem to be inevitable. Division of functions in the maintenance model would permit either federal or state governments to maintain control of access to benefit dollars even if they are not involved in direct management.

8

Objectives and Standards in Long-Term Care

The FSP was conceived with conventional assumptions regarding long-term care objectives. It was assumed that both the public interest in expenditure control and the private preferences of older disabled persons would be served by an effort to prevent unnecessary institutionalization. If successful, the project would demonstrate that the provision of modest assistance to families would lead to reductions in rates of institutionalization among older persons with serious functional disabilities. As a corollary, the savings in reduced institutional care expenditures would offset the costs of assistance to family caretakers.

The analysis of data on the problems that brought families to the program, the nature of the assistance offered, and the reactions of families has led to a reexamination of conventionally accepted assumptions and objectives for long-term care. To amend the perceived flaws, an alternative formulation emphasizing quality-of-life circumstances is recommended.

General Long-Term Care Objectives

Rapidly increasing public expenditures for nursing-home care and the preference of the elderly for independent living arrangements provide a basic argument for community-based long-term care.[1] A closer analysis, however, reveals serious problems with these rationales. Public officials seeking to control institutional care expenditures can intervene more directly by setting tighter limits on the number of long-term care beds they authorize. Conscientiously administered screening and strict entry criteria can also limit publicly financed institutional care. Such strategies, of course, can lead to increased discharge problems for acute-care hospitals and to prolonged hospitalization of marginal long-term care patients. Stricter limits on reimbursement for patients awaiting alternate care, however, can put greater pressure on hospitals to discharge patients to independent living arrangements regardless of the consequences for patients.

Even if the cost per case of home care is less than institutional care and home care is substituted to some extent for institutional care, an aggregate expansion of service is likely to lead to a net increase in public expenditures. For every institutionalized older person, there are two or three comparably disabled being cared for by their families.[2] Subsidized home care will be attractive to families who would not have used institutional care. The arguments against excluding disabled elderly with families from service were presented earlier.

Public savings experienced through reduced use of institutional care are likely to be more than offset by increases in the total number of individuals and families participating in publicly financed long-term care.

The provision of home care for those unable to maintain themselves is expected to reduce mortality and promote longevity. The importance that the public attaches to the continuation of life is reflected in outcries against occasionally publicized accounts of the elderly who die alone and unattended at home. The care provided in nursing homes generally allows the disabled to survive, but there is public concern about the quality of the life that is prolonged. Mere survival is an insufficient objective. It must be supplemented with other objectives that address the circumstances under which people live.

Long-term care generally is thought to include both maintenance and restorative service.[3] Optimal functioning and a return to independent living are placed within the domain of long-term care objectives. These are traditional objectives for the health care, physical and occupational therapies, and special education offered to the handicapped. If chronic impairment is a condition of eligibility, then rehabilitation and restoration of functioning is unrealistic. Long-term care cannot be expected to have any direct effect on functioning, not even on decelerating deterioration.

Since illness or injury often leads to the need for long-term care, conventional curative and restorative objectives must be included in the configuration. Because loss of functioning may be permanent, substantial conventional health objectives may be only partially achieved and on a delayed basis. Long-term care is concerned with the enduring consequences of illness or injury. More is needed than the conventional health objectives of curing, restoring, and rehabilitating.

Maximization of choice and minimization of restriction belong in the configuration of long-term care objectives. Community-based long-term care is justified in part on the basis of consumer preference. Critics note the restrictive qualities of institutional life and argue that it tends to encourage unnecessary dependence. In addition, individual freedom is valued in American society. To the extent feasible, therefore, long-term care should be provided in a manner that minimizes the restrictions experienced by recipients. Freedom can also be interpreted as the presence of opportunity. Some evaluate long-term care on the basis of the opportunities it provides for the functionally disabled. They presume the functionally disabled to be better off when allowed choices.[4] For the choice to be real, however, the functionally disabled and their agents must be aware of their alternatives and be able to select from among them on an informed basis.

Although the maximization of options is a useful objective in long-term care, the quality of options is also important. A choice between two attractive options is preferable to a choice between two unattractive ones. For example, in a choice between residential settings, both institutional and home settings should present positive qualities. Long-term care objectives should include both maximization of choice and maximization of the quality of the various alternatives.

The enhancement of the mental well-being of the disabled person sometimes is suggested as a long-term care objective.[5] Unfortunately there are important, fundamental problems with morale and life satisfaction as objectives for maintenance aspects of long-term care. Part of the difficulty is inherent in their measurement. As attitudinal variables, morale and life satisfaction cannot be observed directly; they are inferred on the basis of a verbal exchange. Although such measures have been developed that have been found to be reliable when administered in research settings, these measures appear to be highly vulnerable to corruption if they are used regularly as a basis for decision making regarding public programs. For example, response patterns may be affected by respondent awareness of the potential uses of morale data.[6] Some respondents might report artificially low morale as part of a plea for an increase in desired services. Positively exaggerated morale might be reported in other instances as a way of showing appreciation to service providers. Further, service providers aware of the timing of morale measurement might introduce marketing strategies designed to elicit a temporary and artificially inflated level of reported life satisfaction.

In addition, morale and life satisfaction are substantially affected by variables out of the control of long-term care providers. The effects of short-term mood cycles and perception of health upon morale are important illustrations of the difficulty.[7] The functionally disabled often correctly recognize themselves to be in poor health, and their morale is predictably affected negatively by their poor health status. Providers of maintenance care should be asked to deliver services in a pleasing manner, but it does not seem reasonable to expect service providers to be fully accountable for the morale of their clients. Research on forces affecting the morale of the functionally disabled is important in suggesting intervention strategies that maximize contentment. Morale and life satisfaction, however, are less than fully satisfactory as bases for judging the adequacy of long-term care.

An Alternate Formulation

Limitations in objectives commonly proposed for long-term care invite consideration of an alternative that emphasizes the immediate implications of long-term care. In human-service programming, it is always possible to articulate a hierarchy of objectives ranging from the immediately desired consequences of intervention to some ultimately desired results. Typically evaluation evidence is more readily available for immediate rather than ultimate objectives. In evaluating programs, a distinction should be made between basic and bonus objectives. The fundamental worth of a program should be judged on the basic objectives, which must be measurable. Bonus objectives are other outcomes that are desirable but not crucial to program survival. Because they are not critical, greater measurement difficulties can be tolerated.

Long-term care is concerned with the provision of service to persons unable to function independently and to care for themselves. The fundamental purpose of long-term care, then, is to provide the impaired with assistance in tasks of daily living. In some instances, functional disability includes an inability to prepare meals. In this case, a service provider is expected to prepare, deliver, and perhaps serve food. The basic objective is to ensure that the client eats adequately. Functional disability may include an inability to go out to shop for necessary household supplies. Long-term care may involve shopping assistance. In this case, the basic objective is to ensure the presence of basic supplies in the household. Functionally disabled persons may be unable to bathe independently. The service provider offers help with bathing, with the objective being to enable the client to maintain bodily cleanliness. The basic objective is the realization of adequate solutions to daily living problems that follow from the functional deficits of clients.

No attempt is made in this formulation to restrict solutions to daily living problems that can be clearly traced to some specific impairment. Because of the close link between impairment and other environmental, residential, and social variables, the segregation of problems according to cause is artificial. Also, nursing homes currently are expected to meet all of their residents' daily living problems. Similar expectations of community-based care are reasonable.

Measuring Quality of Circumstances

If long-term care is evaluated on the basis of the solutions it produces to problems of daily living, it is essential to specify the problem domain and construct a measurement device. This domain is referred to as "quality of circumstances." The term *quality of life* is not used because it is closely associated with life satisfaction and morale measures.

Description of an individual's life circumstances can be a highly demanding task. Some of the elements of life circumstances are universal; others reflect culture and stage in the life cycle. Attempts to specify the life circumstances of the functionally disabled should be conditioned by explicit assumptions regarding culture and stage in life cycle. Necessarily, resource limitations dictate that any attempt to specify and measure life circumstances will also be incomplete. The following elements might be included in an attempt to describe the circumstances of a functionally disabled older person in contemporary American society:

1. Shelter
    a. Temperature moderation
    b. Toilet facilities
    c. Meal-preparation facilities
    d. Bathing facilities

    e. Sleeping facilities

    f. Safety and security provisions

    g. Privacy

    h. Basic facilities for expressive activities (such as living space and furniture)

    i. Communication facilities (such as a telephone and door bell)

    j. Lighting

    k. Cleanliness

2. Eating patterns

    a. Food intake necessary for nutritional requirements

    b. Expressive aspects of eating

3. Sleeping patterns

    a. Nighttime sleep

    b. Daytime rest

4. Personal care patterns

    a. Toileting

    b. Bathing

    c. Grooming

5. Clothing

    a. Availability of garments appropriate for various weather conditions and social situations

    b. Cleanliness of clothing

6. Activity and self-expression

    a. Exercise

    b. Social contact

    c. Shopping

    d. Use of mass media

    e. Recreational or hobby activities

7. Health maintenance

    a. Access to common self-care resources (such as aspirin, antacid, and bandages)

    b. Access to professional health care

8. Mobility

    a. Within dwelling unit

    b. Outside of dwelling unit

9. Choice

    a. Discretion in timing of daily activities

    b. Discretion in personal attire

    c. Food options

    d. Expressive activity options

The organization of the list admittedly is arbitrary. The list may include more overlap than is desirable. It is not clear, for example, whether mobility should be excluded as a dimension. Mobility might be considered simply as instrumental to other dimensions, notably activity and self-expression. Or mobility may be so basic to a conventional life-style that it should be considered in its own right. Choice cuts across other categories. It is included separately because restrictions on personal discretion are fundamental to the widespread criticism of institutional life.

Sexual expression is not included on the list. Anticipation of measurement difficulties, uncertainties about its salience to the very old, and the marginal role usually assumed by service providers in facilitating sexual expression account for its absence. If care for the young adult disabled were at issue, inclusion of opportunities for sexual expression would be important.

Participation in the world of work is also absent from the list. Gainful employment increasingly is expected of both adult men and women in middle-class American society. It is part of their basic social identity. Such employment is a highly complex matter among the elderly. Many elderly persons continue to be engaged in the world of work; others withdraw voluntarily. Mandatory retirement is a contested public issue. The lack of clear-cut employment expectations for the elderly justifies its exclusion for them. A description of life circumstances for younger adults in American society, however, would have to include employment opportunity and employment participation.

Also excluded from the list is participation in family life. For most persons in American society, participation in a nuclear or extended family is not simply instrumental to personal well-being but so fundamental to their social circumstances that it is valued in its own right. Positive participation in a family or a substitute mutual-support group could be considered central to adult identity in American society. Involvement in a family or other mutual support group could be considered an aspect of quality of circumstances. The complexity of the domain, however, makes it difficult to address. The voluntary aspect of participation in informal support groups is one source of complications. In some instances, participation in family life is oppressive for individuals. Divorce laws, for example, establish the right of individuals to withdraw from unsatisfactory marriages. Mortality introduces complications, particularly among the elderly. Remarriage is not a realistic expectation for many widows and widowers. Ambiguity about public responsibility for enhancement of family life or other informal supports is another source of complication. Thus family life is largely a private matter. The degree to which the public should assume responsibility for creating or enhancing opportunities for family or mutual support-group involvement on the part of the functionally disabled is not clear.

At least from an analytic perspective, an individual's circumstances involve interaction with an environment. Even in a simplified formulation that overlooks the individual's capacity to create and shape opportunities, individuals have an opportunity to respond differentially to various opportunities in their environment. At a minimum, they can decline to respond to opportunity. From an evaluation perspective, both opportunity and response to opportunity may be important. Service providers can be held directly responsible for the provision of opportunities. Ordinarily, however, opportunities are not considered intrinsically valuable. The expectation of at least occasional use of opportunity accounts for the value attached to it. Behavioral response to opportunity is important in understanding the contribution of services to problem solving. A functionally disabled person, for example, needs to eat but may be incapable of meal preparation. A helping agent may prepare and serve a meal to the disabled person. The disabled person given the opportunity to eat the meal, however, can refuse. If the meal is refused, it does not satisfy the need for nutrition. Nonacceptance (refusal) of opportunity invites a number of interpretations: the opportunity was not fully understood, the opportunity was defective, no immediate action was needed, and better problem-solving options were perceived to be available. Positive response to opportunity usually can be interpreted as an indication of at least partial and temporary problem solving. Very high rates of positive response to opportunity, however, should be interpreted cautiously. They may indicate coercion or intimidation.

Response to opportunity is regarded as a behavioral outcome variable. In principle, it can be measured through observation. Although behavioral outcome data are preferred, it may not always be feasible to obtain them. Two examples concerned with shelter illustrate problems. Room temperature is one shelter variable. Ideally standards of adequacy would be set by specifying acceptable temperature ranges. Data would be obtained on actual temperatures. In reality, monitoring of actual temperatures may not be feasible. If it is necessary to obtain temperature information from consumers, there is no assurance that they will be able to report actual temperatures. Instead it may be necessary to rely on their subjective comfort judgments.

Cleanliness is another shelter feature that is useful in illustrating measurement problems. In principle, a standard of adequacy for shelter cleanliness could be established. Conceivably the degree to which the standard is met could be determined through a careful household inspection. In reality, such inspections might be excessively time-consuming, and the public might not tolerate the inconvenience and intrusion. In the absence of a measure of actual cleanliness, an evaluation researcher might have to rely either on a process measure such as reported frequency of cleaning activity or a subjective outcome measure such as client satisfaction with household cleanliness.

Tables 8-1 and 8-2 illustrate measurement instrument formats for aspects of quality of circumstances. In the simpler form (table 8-1), information on shelter is solicited. Two examples are offered concerned with shelter. One shelter aspect addresses the presence of conventional furnishings. The second is concerned with building security. A privacy domain is concerned with the physical means of separation from others during the day and at night.

In its more complex form, the instrument (table 8-2) differentiates among possible adverse impact of disability upon an activity area, opportunity to engage in an activity, and actual activity. For example, an initial disability impact

Table 8–1
Simple Measurement Instrument Format

Domain	Circumstances
Shelter: furniture	Do the furnishings of your apartment include: A bed for you? A chair in which you can regularly sit? A chair in which another person can sit? A table on which meals can be served? A curtain or shade over the window in your sleeping area?
Shelter: security	Do you have a lock that works on all outside doors? Do you have a way of seeing or speaking with persons at your door before you let them in?
Privacy	Do you usually have a room available during the day in which you can be alone? Do you have a room in which you sleep that is private or that you share only with your spouse?

question is concerned with the respondent's ability to see well enough to read a newspaper. Those who respond affirmatively are asked if they can get a newspaper daily if they desire. Those reporting visual difficulties are asked about the availability of a person to read the newspaper aloud. In the activity category, respondents are asked how often they read a newspaper or listen if it is read to them. A second example concerns shopping. Information is sought about the respondent's ability to go shopping with or without a companion. For both conditions, information is sought on how often it is possible to go shopping. Finally information is sought on the actual number of shopping trips taken in the previous week.

Standards in Community-Based Long-Term Care

It is one matter to describe the circumstances of a person and another to characterize their quality because quality implies a judgment about the value, adequacy, or desirability of circumstances. This formulation leads, then, to questions about the authority and basis for setting standards and the means of monitoring or regulating compliance with standards.

Legislators, employees of public regulatory agencies, health and welfare professionals, courts, relatives of the functionally disabled, and the functionally disabled themselves are all potential judges of the adequacy of circumstances. Since legislators have the responsibility of authorizing assistance programs for the functionally disabled and raising tax revenues to finance assistance, they

Table 8–2
Complex Measurement Instrument Format

Domain	Disability Impact	Opportunity	Activity
Mass media (newspaper)	Are you able to see well enough to read a newspaper? ___Yes ___No If yes: _____ If no: _____	Can you get a newspaper to read everyday if you want to? ___Yes ___No Is there someone who will read a newspaper to you if you want? ___Never ___Once or twice a week ___Three or four times ___Five or six times a week ___Every day	In the past week, how often did you read a newspaper or have one read to you? ___Not at all ___Once or twice ___Three or four times ___Five or six times ___Every day
Shopping	Are you able to get around well enough so that you can go out shopping alone? ___Yes ___No If yes: _____ If no: _____ Can you go shopping if you have someone to go along with you? ___No ___Yes If yes: _____	When the weather is good is there anything which keeps you from going out shopping every day? ___No ___Yes If no: _____ If yes: _____ How often is it possible for you to go out shopping? ___Never ___Less than once a week ___Once or twice a week ___3 to 6 times a week ___At least once a day	In the past week, how often have you actually gone out shopping? ___Not at all ___Once or twice ___3 or 4 times ___5 or 6 times ___Every day

might be entitled to define adequacy. It is most unlikely, however, that legislators would attend to the level of detail required in establishing quality-of-circumstance standards for the functionally disabled. Legislative bodies characteristically authorize programs with broad purposes and delegate such matters as the development of standards to administrative agencies. Legislative bodies attach monetary amounts to programs, but they are not close to the day-to-day quality of services delivered. Employees of regulatory agencies may be asked to formulate standards on the basis of their professional expertise. For services that require the specialized knowledge and skills presumably concentrated within a professional group, a strong argument can be made for professional dominance in standard setting. Care of the functionally disabled, however, does not require professional expertise. To the extent that care is provided at public expense, it seems appropriate that standards of care should reflect general societal values. The extent to which employees of public agencies who formulate standards reflect societal values is unknown.

Professionals who directly serve the functionally disabled might be asked to represent the larger society in establishing standards on a case-by-case basis. A number of problems can be anticipated, however, that limit the value of this approach. In their preoccupation with their area of expertise, some professionals, notably physicians, may be insensitive to quality-of-circumstance issues, and they may vary a great deal among one another in interpreting community values.[8] In addition, some professionals may be more responsive to client demands than to their own interpretation of general community values. For example, clients of the FSP varied greatly in the extent of care they willingly provided before seeking help. Other consumers also vary greatly in the vigor and intensity with which they appeal for help and complain about quality of assistance. Under these circumstances, serious inequities can be expected in the scope of assistance received by the functionally disabled.

Courts might assume standard-setting responsibilities. If consumer advocates persuade the courts that neither legislative nor administrative bodies will establish and enforce a reasonable standard of adequacy, the courts may do so. There are several precedents for such an approach. The New York State Willowbrook consent decree is one example.[9] A federal judge ruled that conditions in a public institution on Staten Island for the retarded were intolerable. In response, the court established highly specific standards regarding circumstances that residents of that institution should experience, not only in the institution but in the more-normal settings to which they would be transferred eventually. Further, the court created a panel authorized to monitor residential settings on their compliance with the standards recommended by a group of professionals. Although the court had authority to act on this matter, questions may be raised about the extent to which the values reflected in the decision were consistent with those of the larger society. Because of cost concerns, New York State has not implemented the decree as fully and rapidly as the court desired.

Alternately, the problem of establishing standards for circumstances of the functionally disabled might be addressed by establishing client satisfaction as the major objective for long-term care. The functionally disabled might be surveyed regarding the degree of their satisfaction with their own circumstances. Although consumer satisfaction would appear to be important as an aspect of long-term care objectives, it is not by itself fully satisfactory as an objective. Policy makers have reason to be concerned that the functionally disabled, like other interest groups, may be unreasonable in making escalating demands. In time they might set their satisfaction threshold so high that policy makers would not find it feasible to make sufficient resources available. Further, the sensitivity of satisfaction measures to spurious and superficial forces tends to detract from the utility of satisfaction as a basis for quality standards.

Policy makers may be forced, then, to retreat to quality of circumstances as a more-proximate outcome variable. It may be feasible for public programs to ensure circumstances qualitatively consistent with standards when it is not feasible to ensure consumer satisfaction. The functionally disabled might be consulted in the formulation of standards. Because standards should reflect general community values and resource limitations, it is unlikely that the formulation of standards would be left to the functionally disabled alone.

Another potential basis for establishing quality-of-circumstance standards is to use each functionally disabled person as his or her own standard. When the functional disability was of recent origin, this approach would be applicable. The goal would be to enable the individual to approximate the life-style enjoyed before the onset of the disabling condition. For a person losing the capacity to walk, for example, an attempt might be made to sustain the individual's mobility opportunities. But a number of limitations are evident in the use of the functionally disabled as their own standard. The approach does not apply to those with functional disability of congenital origins, and when disabilities are of very long duration, pre-onset life patterns may lose their pertinence since life-style expectations are affected by stage in the life cycle and societal trends. In addition, valid data on consumer circumstance prior to onset may be difficult to obtain. Beyond recall problems, service applicants may give exaggerated accounts of their former circumstances if they have reason to believe it will add to the scope of assistance they receive. The approach also does not specify the extent to which the disabled person should be expected to approximate a previous life pattern.

Implicit in an approach that uses each disabled person as his or her own standard is an assumption that ameliorative intervention for the functionally disabled should not have implications for resource redistribution. In fact, public services for the functionally disabled may call attention to persons who have experienced highly deprived life circumstances prior to the onset of disability because of poverty. A return to such circumstances may be regarded as offensive by the professional persons involved. They may believe that in some cases institutional placement for the functionally disabled is preferable to extremely poor living conditions that preceded the onset of the disability.[10] Under some circumstances, then, alleviation of poverty may be important as a secondary objective in long-term care. If it is impractical or undesirable to use the functionally disabled as their own standard, life-styles prevailing among the nondisabled of similar age and sex might be employed in establishing standards of circumstances for the functionally disabled. Empirical data on life-styles among the nondisabled, therefore, would be useful as a base against which the circumstances of the disabled might be judged.

An issue in all attempts to establish quality-of-circumstance objectives is that impairments may set limits on what is possible in various aspects of life-style. Total blindness, for example, rules out visual experiences, but other sensory experiences can be introduced as a partial substitute. Somehow quality-of-circumstance standards must reflect limits set by impairments.

If the adequacy of public response to the needs of the functionally disabled is to be judged on the basis of the quality of their circumstances, however, it would be desirable if the judgments were based on explicit standards. Since no fully satisfactory vehicle for formulating such standards currently exists, a new institutional vehicle might be created to assume the standard-setting responsibility. The public agency with primary responsibility for the care of the functionally disabled might authorize the formation of citizen groups at a community level whose charge would be to establish quality-of-circumstance standards. The groups would be expected to reflect general community standards in judging the degree to which it is important for the functionally disabled to approximate generally prevailing standards on various life-style dimensions. The citizen groups would also be expected to reflect community concerns about implications of publicly financed services for taxes. The role of these groups would be similar to that which community school boards play in balancing interests in the quality of the educational environment and the control of taxes. Local draft boards provide further precedent for the approach suggested here. When they were active, draft boards were a vehicle through which local citizen groups made judgments about individual cases on the basis of federal regulations and military personnel requirements.

The local citizen groups would be asked to review the various dimensions of quality of circumstances and make overall judgments about the importance of various qualitative features. The public agencies with care responsibilities would use the standards in addressing the care needs of functionally disabled individuals. Presumably the citizen panels would seek statistical data on the extent to which the quality of circumstances of the functionally disabled in the community were consistent with its standards. In a weak structural framework, the citizen group could do little more than comment publicly on the degree to which actual conditions were consistent with standards. In a stronger framework, the standard-setting group would have some authority to insist on ameliorative action when serious shortcomings in conditions were observed.

Notes

1. William G. Bell, "Community Care for the Elderly: An Alternative to Institutionalization," *Gerontologist* 13, no. 3 (1973): 349–354.

2. Maureen Baltay, *Long-Term Care for the Elderly and the Disabled* (Washington, D.C.: Congressional Budget Office, (1977) ; and "The Well-Being

of Older People in Cleveland, Ohio" (Washington, D.C.: General Accounting Office, 19 April, 1977).

3. Martin Bloom, "Evaluation Instruments: Tests and Measurements in Long-Term Care," in *Long-Term Care: A Handbook for Researchers, Planners, and Providers,* ed. Sylvia Sherwood (New York: Spectrum Publications, Inc., 1975).

4. For a general discussion of expansion of choice as a social-service objective, see Martin Rein, *Social Policy: Issues of Choice and Change* (New York: Random House, 1970).

5. Sherwood, Sylvia (ed.) *Long-Term Care: A Handbook for Researchers, Planners, and Providers.* (New York: Spectrum Publications, Inc., 1975).

6. Donald Campbell, "Keeping the Data Honest in the Experimenting Society," in *Interdisciplinary Dimensions of Accounting for Social Goals and Social Organizations.* (Columbus, Ohio: Grid, 1977): 37–76.

7. Erdman Palmore and C. Leikart, "Health and Social Factors Related to Life Satisfaction," *Journal of Health and Social Behavior* 13 (1972): 58–80; J. Edwards and D. Klemnack, "Correlates of Life Satisfaction: A Re-Examination," *Journal of Gerontology* 28, no. 4 (1973): 497–502; and Elmer Spreitzer and Eldon E. Snyder, "Correlates of Life Satisfaction Among the Aged," *Journal of Gerontology* 29, no. 4 (1974): 457–458.

8. B.M. Braginsky et al. *Message of Madness: The Mental Hospital as a Last Resort* (New York: Holt, Rinehart & Winston, 1969).

9. (Willowbrook Consent Judgment) *New York State Association for Retarded Citizens and Parisi* v. *Carey*, 357 F. Supp. 752, 756 (E.D.N.Y. 1973), approved 393 F. Supp. 715 (E.D.N.Y. 1975), affirmed on appeal 596 F. 2d 27 (2nd Cir. Ct. of Appeals, 1979).

10. William J. Foley, U.S. Menger, and D.P. Schneider. "A Comparison of the Level of Care Predictions of Six Long-Term Care Patient Assessment Systems," *American Journal of Public Health* 70, no. 1 (1980): 1152–1161.

Appendix: Research and Evaluation Method

This study employs an exploratory-longitudinal design. Families were observed shortly after the introduction of service and at one year intervals for as long as they remained in service. A sample of interviews was also conducted when clients' services were terminated. Research questions (see chapter 2) focused on the role of the family as service agent, its structure and functions, its adaptation to formally organized assistance, and its persistence in service when supported by an outside agency.

In order to detect the subtlety in provider-and-client negotiations over service and observe variation in administrative handling of cases, a qualitative approach was required. The continuation of families in service also created an opportunity for repeated observations and therefore a need for more standardized assessments. The result of these circumstances and opportunities is a combination of both structured and unstructured sources of data.

Twelve of the ninety-six families in the original sample terminated from the program during the first year. Four of the elderly persons died and two were placed in nursing homes in the first year. Three of the elderly moved out of the program's catchment area, and three families were found to be uncooperative or the service agreement broke down. Of the eighty-four families who were interviewed after one year of FSP services, twenty-five terminated from the program during the second year and eleven families had not been in service up to two years when research staff stopped interviewing family members. Of the twenty-five terminations in the second year, nine of the elderly persons died and ten had been placed in nursing homes. Four of the elderly moved out of the program catchment area and service agreement broke down with two families.

The initial face-to-face interview was with the primary family member providing care. The Functioning for Independent Living Scale (FIL) was administered. The instrument itself is reproduced in this appendix. The FIL scale was modeled after other instruments known to obtain reliable data on functional impairments. Qualitative descriptions of the older person's condition were recorded. The initial interview also focused on the family's first experiences with the FSP. Family members were asked how they learned about the program, how the program was described to them by the social worker, which services they may have requested, and which services were offered by the program. They were then asked about their own motivation for family care, the impact of these responsibilities on their own lives, and the difficult aspects and possible satisfactions related to caring for an elderly relative. Finally, the activities of other family members were assessed and the family member's concern about the future course of care was discussed.

   Although the FSP social workers were not formally interviewed, interviewers consulted the case record to get basic information about the family,
the older person, the early stages of service negotiation, and the FSP services
being provided. The interviewers also consulted case records before the follow-
up interview in each year.

   In both the first and second year follow-up interviews, the primary supporting family members were asked similar questions. First, both the quantitative
rating on the FIL scale and the qualitative description of the older person's
condition were recorded with a focus on changes that may have taken place
since the last interview. The primary supporting relatives were asked about any
accidents, falls, hospitalizations, and changes in the medical condition of the
elderly relative.

   Changes in family support and FSP services were also assessed from year to
year. Changes in the level of support provided by both the primary supporting
relative and the family network were noted, as well as the reasons for changes.
Supporting relatives were asked about possible changes in the actual services
from FSP and other service providers, such as changes in the hours or cost of
homemaker service, or the initiation of other public entitlements to service.
Finally, the primary supporting relatives were asked about the continuing impact
of the disability and outside assistance upon them and their families.

   In addition to the initial and follow-up interviews, a special questionnaire
was sent to primary supporting family members to elicit the overall amount and
types of activities they performed for the elderly person. This questionnaire
covered the major activities that families could perform for the elderly such as
shopping, light housekeeping, home repairs, personal care, assistance with
transfers, financial assistance, and so on. The form is reproduced in table A-1.
This family-activities questionnaire was sent to seventy-four family members
during the course of the program. Fifty-five of the families were sent two
questionnaires. In the second questionnaire they were asked to report their
activities *before* FSP services were initiated.

   Data from the initial interview, the first and second year follow-up interview, and the family-activities questionnaire were coded and processed into
SPSS system files.

Functioning for Independent Living Scale

  I. Vision   *SCORE*
     A. Sees well enough with or without glasses to
         recognize all common household objects
         and/or to negotiate street crossings   _____   0
     B. Sees well enough with or without glasses to
         recognize *most* household objects but cannot
         discriminate well enough to read labels on
         common objects   _____   2

SCORE

C. Sees well enough with or without glasses to recognize *most* household objects but cannot see well enough to negotiate street crossings   _____   2

D. Sees well enough with or without glasses to recognize *most* household objects but cannot see well enough to discriminate among labels on common objects or to negotiate street crossings   _____   4

E. Does not see well enough with or without glasses to recognize most household objects   _____   5

II. Hearing and Speech

A. Speech and hearing with or without mechanical aid adequate to permit essential conversation   _____   0

B. Speech is adequate to permit essential conversation but hearing with or without mechanical aid is not   _____   2

C. Hearing is adequte with or without mechanical aid to permit essential understanding but speech is not adequate for essential conversation   _____   2

D. Neither speech nor hearing with or without mechanical aid is adequate to permit essential conversation   _____   4

III. Mobility

A. Able to walk outdoors up to eight blocks and climb one flight of stairs   _____   0

B. Able to walk outdoors but can walk no more than one block   _____   1

C. Able to walk outdoors up to eight blocks but unable to climb one flight of stairs   _____   1

D. Able to walk outdoors no more than one block and unable to climb one flight of stairs   _____   2

E. Able to move about freely within single-floor dwelling unit without mechanical assistance (for example, wheelchair or walker). Unable to walk outdoors or climb one flight of stairs   _____   3

F. Able to move about freely within single-floor dwelling unit only with mechanical assistance. Unable to walk outdoors or climb one flight of stairs   _____   4

G. Not able to move about freely within single-floor dwelling unit even with mechanical assistance. Unable to walk outdoors or climb one flight of stairs   _____   6

IV. Transfer   *SCORE*
   A.   Able to enter and leave bed, chair,
       toilet, bath (or shower), and automobile
       independently   _____   0
   B.   *Unable* to enter and leave independently:

       Bed_____4 Chair_____3

       Toilet _____ 2 Bath or shower_____2   (Divide
                                                  total
                                                 score
       Automobile_____ 1   _____ by 2)

V. Hand and Arm Movement
   A.   Able to reach for, grasp, lift, and
       manipulate common household objects   _____   0
   B.   Able to reach for, grasp, lift, and
       manipulate common household objects
       except items lighter and more delicate
       than a pencil   _____   2
   C.   Able to reach for, grasp, lift, and
       manipulate common household objects
       except items weighing more than
       five pounds   _____   2
   D.   Unable to handle small or heavy objects.
       Regular difficulty with some objects or
       even intermediate size and weight   _____   4
   E.   Unable to reach for, grasp, lift, and
       manipulate most common household
       objects   _____   6

VI. Bowel and Bladder Control
   A.   Controls urination and bowel movement
       completely by self   _____   0
   B.   Has occasional urinary accidents   _____   1
   C.   Has occasional bowel accidents   _____   2
   D.   Has frequent urinary accidents   _____   3
   E.   Incontinent   _____   6

VII. Confused Behavior
   Memory
   A.   Remembers to prepare meals, keep
       appointments, and/or take medication
       if occasionally reminded   _____   0
   B.   Occasionally forgets to prepare meals,
       keep appointments, and/or take
       medication   _____   1

VII. Confused Behavior (contd.)

SCORE

C. Cannot remember to prepare meals, keep appointments, and/or take medication without constant supervision _____ 2

Identity

A. Always remembers own name and address and can give them when requested _____ 0

B. On at least one occasion was unable to remember name and/or address _____ 1

C. Regularly forgets name and/or address _____ 2

Speech

A. Is able to spontaneously communicate thoughts and intentions in a way that the listener can always understand _____ 0

B. Speaks infrequently. Speech is confused but can be understood by a patient, careful listener _____ 1

C. Rarely speaks spontaneously and/or speech is incoherent _____ 2

Wandering

A. Can leave place of residence and return without getting lost _____ 0

B. Cannot be alone on the street without getting lost. Requires assistance getting home _____ 2

C. Must be supervised continuously or will wander away from residence and become lost _____ 4

Non-Conventional Behavior

A. Dresses appropriately, maintains personal hygiene, cooperates with the family's support plan _____ 0

B. Occasionally requires instruction on dress and hygiene and/or resists essential assistance _____ 2

C. Requires daily instruction on dress and hygiene and/or regularly disrupts the family's support plan _____ 4

Table A-1
Family Activity Scale

These service activities are performed currently on behalf of the disabled family member by persons identified by the following initials: Sn = son, D = daughter, B = brother, SS = sister, M = mother, F = father, S-1 = son-in-law, O = other relative, D-1 = daughter-in law, F = friend or neighbor, Sp = spouse, Gs = grandson, Gd = granddaughter.

Items	(1) At Least Once a Day	(2) 3 or 4 Times a Week	(3) 1 or 2 Times a Week	(4) 1 to 3 Times a Month	(5) Less Than Once a Month	(6) Never or Not Applicable
Go shopping for personal items and food, etc.	___	___	___	___	___	___
Prepare meals	___	___	___	___	___	___
Do light housecleaning (for example, dust, wash dishes, or take out trash)	___	___	___	___	___	___
Do heavy housecleaning (for example, scrub floors, wash windows, or move furniture)	___	___	___	___	___	___
Arrange for or make home repairs (for example, heating, plumbing, painting)	___	___	___	___	___	___
Administer or supervise medication	___	___	___	___	___	___

Help with laundry

Supervise or assist with grooming, personal hygiene or dress (for example, bathing, toileting, clothes selection)

Assist with transfer (for example, moving from bed to chair, or from toilet to chair)

Sometimes contribute money for expenses

Help manage finances (for example, cash the Social Security check, or keep the bank account)

Assist in transportation by escorting in a car, taxi, or on public transportation

Assist in physical exercise program (for example, physical therapy or accompany on walks)

Substitute for the temporarily absent caregiver in order to assure the continual presence of a responsible person

Index

About the Authors

Dwight L. Frankfather is assistant professor at the University of Chicago School of Social Service Administration. His teaching and research concern services for the chronically mentally ill and physically impaired. Dr. Frankfather received the M.S.W. and Ph.D. from the Heller School for Advanced Studies in Social Welfare, Brandeis University.

Michael J. Smith is assistant professor at the Hunter College School of Social Work, where he is engaged in the study of social-welfare policy and family structure. Dr. Smith is a graduate of Columbia University, School of Social Work.

Francis G. Caro is the director of the Institute for Social Welfare Research at the Community Service Society of New York. Dr. Caro specializes in the areas of program evaluation and long-term-care research and is currently directing a large-scale evaluation of home care in New York City. He is a graduate of the University of Minnesota with a doctorate in sociology.